A PRACTICAL GUIDE TO
3D ULTRASOUND

A PRACTICAL GUIDE TO 3D ULTRASOUND

Reem S. Abu-Rustum, MD

Director, Center For Advanced Fetal Care
Tripoli, Lebanon

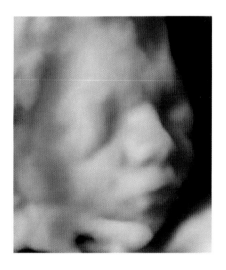

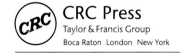

CRC Press
Taylor & Francis Group
Boca Raton London New York

CRC Press is an imprint of the
Taylor & Francis Group, an **informa** business

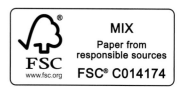

CRC Press
Taylor & Francis Group
6000 Broken Sound Parkway NW, Suite 300
Boca Raton, FL 33487-2742

© 2015 by Taylor & Francis Group, LLC
CRC Press is an imprint of Taylor & Francis Group, an Informa business

No claim to original U.S. Government works

Printed on acid-free paper
Version Date: 20141023

International Standard Book Number-13: 978-1-4822-1433-8 (Paperback)

Visit the Taylor & Francis Web site at
http://www.taylorandfrancis.com

and the CRC Press Web site at
http://www.crcpress.com

This book is dedicated to
All the "perfect imperfections",
The fetuses scanned through the years...
and
To those through whom I came
And those who through me came
With eternal love and appreciation...

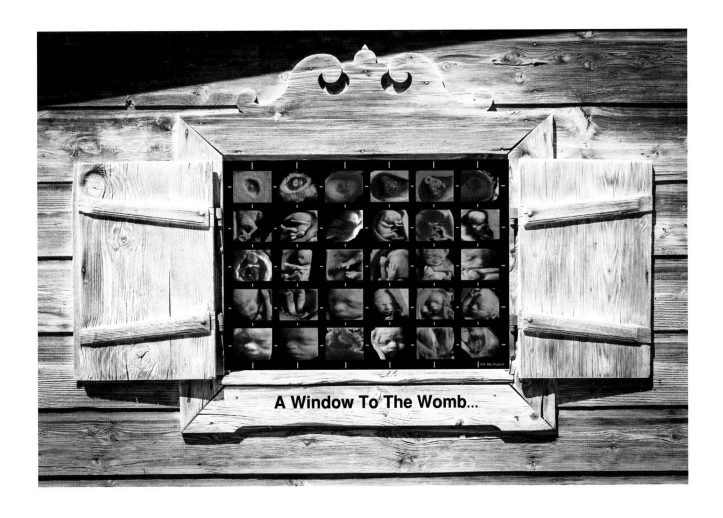

A Window To The Womb...

Contents

Foreword

Three-dimensional (3D) ultrasound was introduced to the medical community over 20 years ago when investigators in Europe and North America reported imaging fetal and gynecological structures. In 2001 I purchased my first 3D/4D ultrasound machine for clinical use and began an exciting journey incorporating this technology into my clinical practice. For the past 13 years 3D/4D technology has advanced to a point that it is indispensable for the serious clinician who performs obstetrical, gynecological, and fetal echocardiographic examinations.

As a result of this technology, there has been an explosion of diagnostic tools, new terminology and concepts that have required the practice of diagnostic ultrasound to be at a high level of commitment by the physician/sonographer providing ultrasound services to patients. While 3D/4D ultrasound is an exciting imaging modality, most of the medical literature relating to this technology focuses on diagnostic results, with few articles addressing how to use the technology. A comparison might be made when years ago travelers were told of the benefits of flying great distances by airplane, but did not understand that an experienced pilot was necessary for this to be accomplished!

This textbook, *A Practical Guide to 3D Ultrasound*, created by Dr. Reem S. Abu-Rustum, helps fill this important void. The chapters contain clear instructions on how to image fetal as well as gynecological structures. The beautiful images provided by the author are perhaps the most compelling part of the textbook. The high quality of the images and the clarity of the instructions contained within the text underscore the experience of Dr. Abu-Rustum in the 3D/4D ultrasound arena. This book will benefit both the novice as well as the experienced physician/sonographer who uses 3D/4D technology in obstetrics and gynecological imaging.

Greggory R. DeVore, MD
Clinical Professor
Department of Obstetrics and Gynecology
David Geffen School of Medicine at UCLA
Los Angeles, California, USA

Director of the Fetal Diagnostic Centers
Pasadena, Tarzana, and Lancaster, California, USA

Director of Perinatology
Providence Tarzana Medical Center
Tarzana, California, USA

Preface

A Practical Guide to 3D Ultrasound was conceived with the beginner in volume sonography in mind. Having decided to venture into this new world with added depth 10 years ago, I felt overwhelmed by all the terminology and the techniques being used. Subsequently, I attended several courses and had the honor of visiting many labs examining all the basics in order to decide what would be of utmost utility in my daily clinical practice. As a result of this exposure to the experts, as well as a review of the clinically applicable literature, this guide was put forth. It is by no means comprehensive, but aims at summarizing all the basics in a concise and practical manner, so that it can be used as an introduction to ease the transition into the third dimension.

I wish to acknowledge Drs. Amelia Cruz, Patrick Duff, and Douglas Richards, who first handed me the transducer, and Dr. Kypros Nicolaides for sparking my interest in fetal medicine. I also wish to recognize the tremendous impact that the work of Drs. Alfred Abuhamad, Beryl Benacerraf, Bernard Benoit, Rabih Chaoui and Greggory DeVore has had on my practice and on the birth of this guide; their pioneering work has served as a constant source of inspiration over the years.

I am forever indebted to the wind that propelled me forward and the sun that lit my professional path, Dr. Keith Stone.

This guide would not have been written had it not been for the unconditional love and support of my lifelong motivator, mentor and guide, my father Dr. Sameer Abu-Rustum, my mother Lina, my husband Kamil, my children Maria and Karim, and my sister Mira; they all believed in me and encouraged me over the years to persevere and complete this project despite many challenges.

In addition, I wish to express my gratitude to Dr. Greggory DeVore for his invaluable guidance and constructive critique of this guide. Last but not least, I thank my editor, Mr. Robert Peden, who saw the value of this project when I approached him with my ambitious proposal; without his backing, this guide would not have been possible. I also thank Ms. Kate Nardoni for all her meticulous work in putting this guide together.

May this guide maximize the utility of your volume sonography, enabling you to feel more secure in your diagnostic capabilities and better able to reassure your patients as to the health of the future generations.

Reem S. Abu-Rustum, MD
Center for Advanced Fetal Care
Tripoli, Lebanon

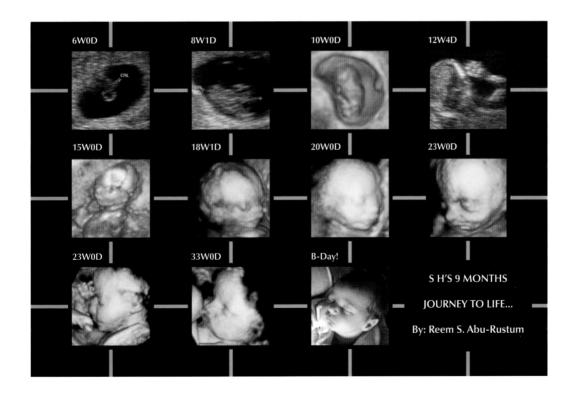

1 Terminology and Basics

INTRODUCTION

Welcome to the world of volume sonography, a world with added depth that enables you to obtain planes previously unattainable using conventional two-dimensional (2D) sonography. In volume sonography, the concept of the "voxel" replaces the "pixel," where you now have three intersecting orthogonal or perpendicular planes with which you are working—the X, Y, and Z planes (Figure 1.1). Where these three planes intersect is the "reference dot," an identifiable, locatable point of interest that can be defined through its relationship within the three planes. Within any acquired three-dimensional (3D) volume is an infinite number of planes, stacked on top of each other, and containing within it all the information needed to analyze that specific area or organ of interest (Figure 1.2). For example, in the first trimester, a volume of the entire fetus may be obtained for analysis at any subsequent point in the future (Abu-Rustum et al. 2012). This volume, if obtained correctly, contains all the planes needed for a full evaluation of the first-trimester fetus (Figure 1.3). This also applies to a volume of the fetal heart that contains within it all the anatomic planes necessary for a complete assessment of the fetal heart and vessels (Abuhamad 2004). Once the volume of data is obtained and stored, it can subsequently be reformatted, post-processed, and displayed interchangeably in the multiplanar (Figure 1.4), surface-rendering mode (Figure 1.5), or in any other mode at any given point in the future.

BASIC CONCEPTS IN THE MULTIPLANAR MODE

1. Marker dot: reference dot
2. Address of the marker dot is determined by the intersection of the X, Y, Z axes (Figure 1.6)

The cornerstone of volume sonography is formed by three main concepts. These are addressed individually in the subsequent chapters.

BASIC CONCEPTS IN VOLUME SONOGRAPHY

1. Volume acquisition
2. Volume manipulation
3. Volume display: multiplanar or rendered

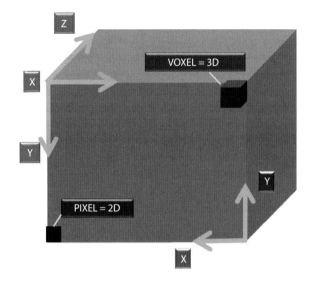

FIGURE 1.1 A cubic volume illustrating the three orthogonal planes along the X, Y, and Z axes, representative of an acquired 3D volume. At the bottom left-hand corner is a 2D rectangle along the X and Y axes, illustrating the 2D concept of a pixel. On the top right is a 3D rectangle along the X, Y, and Z axes, demonstrating the 3D concept of a voxel.

TERMINOLOGY

With volume sonography, there is a new vocabulary to learn (Table 1.1). Some of these terms are generic and others are specific to certain manufacturers. This is why one must become familiar with all the basic terms, their synonyms, and their meanings. It then becomes intuitive as to what is to be used where. The basic concept lies in obtaining what is called a static volume and then visualizing it in the three orthogonal planes in the multiplanar view. If it is subsequently decided to manipulate the volume in order to visualize the image using any of several display modes, this generates the rendered image. This can be surface mode (Figure 1.7), maximal mode (Figure 1.8), minimal mode (Figure 1.9), inversion mode (Figure 1.10), or any combination thereof, to name a few.

ADVANTAGES OF VOLUME SONOGRAPHY

With volume sonography, it is now possible to evaluate planes not previously accessible by 2D ultrasound. In addition, depth perception is now added. The stored volumes are available for educational purposes: they can be utilized for learning anatomy, and they facilitate off-line consultation

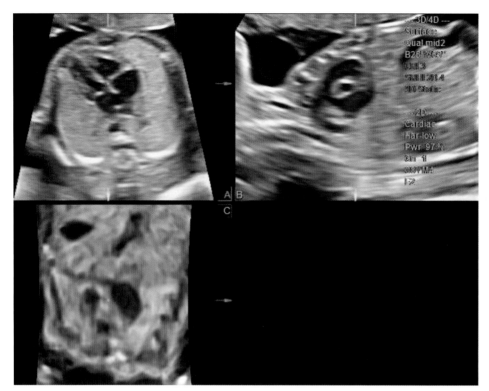

FIGURE 1.2 A 3D volume of the chest of a 22w0d fetus displayed in the multiplanar mode. This volume contains within it all the 2D anatomical planes necessary for a complete assessment of the heart. These 2D planes exist in a defined spatial relationship with respect to each other, and they may be retrieved out of a standardized volume utilizing a specific navigational approach based on the established spatial relationships between them.

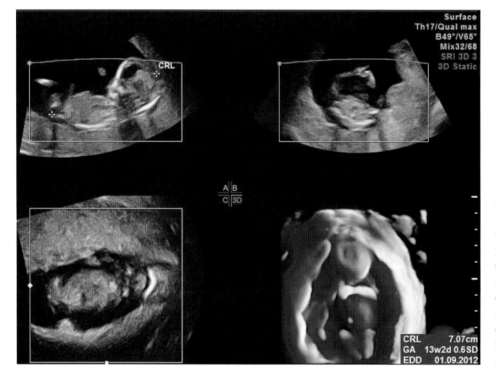

FIGURE 1.3 A 3D volume of a 13w2d fetus depicted in the multiplanar mode (three orthogonal planes A, B, and C) and surface rendered in the bottom right-hand corner, utilizing HD*live*. This volume contains within it all the 2D planes necessary for a complete evaluation of this fetus. These 2D planes may be generated out of the volume by navigation along the three axes.

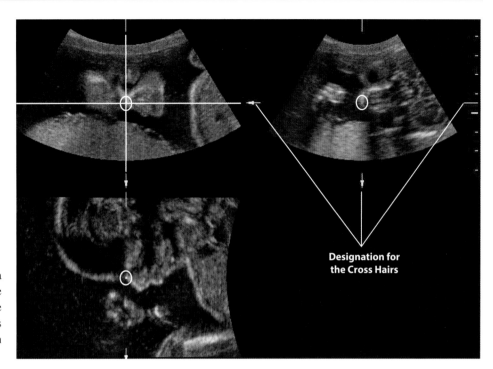

FIGURE 1.4 A 3D volume of a 20w6d fetal face displayed in the three orthogonal planes. Note the position of the reference dot (O). It is the intersection of the cross-hairs in each of the 3 planes.

with experts and over the web. With volume sonography, it is now possible to evaluate such areas as the top of the fetal head, the fetal sutures (Figure 1.11), and the mid-sagittal plane of the fetal head (Figure 1.12). In addition, beam steering allows the visualization of previously unattainable views such as the posterior aspect of structures. As such, the level of a neural tube defect may be localized, and skeletal malformations may be characterized.

Much in terms of fetal behavior can be studied as well by watching fetal movement, awake and sleep cycles, and eyelid movement, all of which further enhance fetal bonding. In gynecologic ultrasound, it is now possible to evaluate the coronal plane of the uterus (Figure 1.13), which enhances sensitivity in the detection of müllerian abnormalities (Bocca et al. 2012; Sakhel et al. 2013). Tumors may be localized more precisely, ovarian cysts may be differentiated from hydrosalpinges, and the tubes may be studied using contrast agents, in addition to facilitating ultrasound-guided biopsies. Volumes may also be rotated 360 degrees to access the back of areas under evaluation. Post-processing tools such as the inversion mode may be applied to highlight areas under examination. This may optimize the visualization of cystic structures (Figure 1.10). Even though there may not be any added diagnostic value to some of these modalities, they certainly help in visual clarification and education, for both physicians and the involved families.

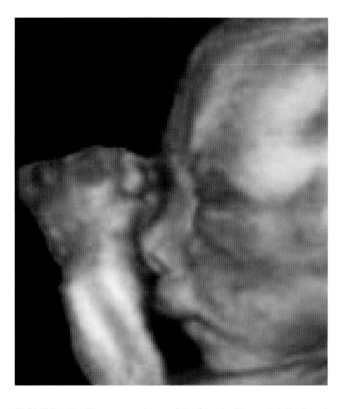

FIGURE 1.5 The same volume of the fetus in Figure 1.4 displayed using surface rendering.

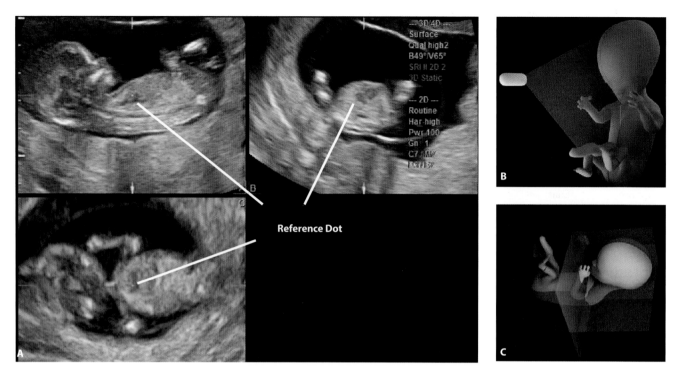

FIGURE 1.6   A 3D volume of a 13w5d fetus. (A) This volume contains within it all the 2D anatomical planes necessary for a complete assessment of the fetus. The reference dot, which is the intersection point of all three orthogonal planes, is placed on the fetal heart. It thus localizes the fetal heart in all three orthogonal planes. (B) A 3D model illustrating the unique acquisition in the first trimester: it is possible to obtain a volume of the entire fetus with a single 3D volume sweep. (C) A 3D model depicting the three intersecting orthogonal planes.

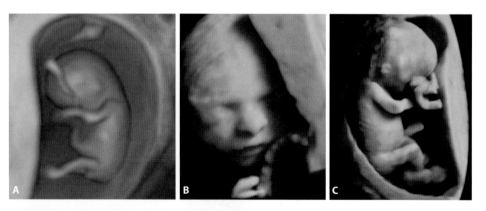

FIGURE 1.7   Samples of 3D surface-rendered volumes depicting the external fetal surface. (A) At 10w5d using dynamic rendering. (B) At 22w2d using HD*live*. (C) At 12w4d using HD*live*.

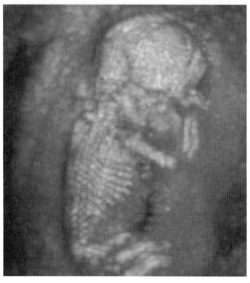

FIGURE 1.8   A 3D volume of a 15w3d fetus displayed in skeletal mode. This modes optimizes the bony structures while minimizing all other gray-scale structures creating an image akin to an x-ray; hence, it is also referred to as x-ray mode.

Table 1.1 **Basic Terminology in Volume Sonography: Synonyms and Clinical Applicability**

Key Word	Synonym	Clinical Applicability
3D Static	2D images, acquired together as part of a volume and displayed in the three orthogonal planes	For evaluating the surface or internal areas of interest
4D	Multiple volumes acquired per second and displayed to depict "3D in motion"	Aids in visualizing fetal movement, facial grimaces, volume of a beating heart
CRI	Compound resolution imaging	Enhances the image resolution
Glass body	Enhanced Doppler information in a gray-scale background	Allows for vascular mapping and studies of vascular structures by minimizing the gray-scale background and highlighting the vascular structure
HD*live*	3D/4D technology with a virtual internal movable light source and sophisticated skin-rendering techniques	Gives a real surface-rendered image of the fetal face and outer surface; may also be used to visualize internal structures and can be combined with other 4D modalities
Inverse mode	Inverts the gray-scale image where the anechoic structures become echogenic and vice versa	Attenuates fluid-filled structures in the fetal brain, heart, gastrointestinal and genitourinary tracts, ovarian pathology, and any other fluid-filled areas
MagiCut	Electronic scalpel with which to sculpt through the volume	Allows volume editing in order to remove access areas and optimize visualization of the area under study
Maximum mode	x-ray mode	Facilitates the study of all bony structures
Minimum mode	Enhances Doppler information while taking out all other gray-scale background information	Highlights the vascular tree and any fluid-filled, anechoic structures; best for evaluation of the heart and fluid-filled structures
OmniView	The "any slice" technique	Allows the slicing of any volume along any line, whether curvilinear or straight, to display hard-to-obtain planes
Reference dot	Marker dot, marker point	The point of intersection of all three orthogonal planes through which rotation along the three axes may be carried out
ROI	Region of interest	Allows the selection of an area of interest within the volume under study which may be viewed in any of four directions
SonoAVC	Automated volume calculator	Allows the automatic selection of fluid-filled areas, color-codes them, and calculates their volume; of maximal utility in ovarian follicular monitoring
SRI	Speckle reduction imaging	Refines the image by reducing the ultrasonographic speckle
STIC	Spatiotemporal image correlation	Enables obtaining and navigating through a volume of a beating heart, with or without color Doppler, throughout one full cardiac cycle
Surface rendering	Image rendering of the fetal surface	Surface topography to visualize the face and external structures; may also be utilized for the internal study of organs
TUI	Tomographic ultrasound imaging	A slicing technique, equivalent to CT, that generates multiple parallel slices, at a user-set distance in mm, of the volume containing an area of interest, facilitating the study of the spatial relationships between structures
VCAD	Volume computer-aided diagnosis	Automatic image retrieval of predefined standardized cardiac planes out of a volume of the fetal heart which may allow a complete examination of the cardiac structures out of the standardized volume
VCI-A and VCI-C	Volume contrast imaging	Allows thick-slice scanning in order to decrease artifacts in either plane A or C; static VCI allows marked improvement in image quality
VOCAL	Virtual organ computer-aided analysis	Volume calculation of areas in question such as ovarian cysts, follicles, urine production, lung mass, and so on, out of an acquired volume

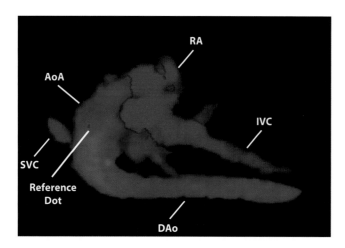

FIGURE 1.9 A 3D volume of a 33-week fetus displayed in minimal mode. This volume utilizes color Doppler and depicts the aortic arch (AoA) where the red reference dot is, descending aorta (DAo), as well as the right atrium (RA) with the superior and inferior venae cavae (SVC, IVC).

Perhaps one of the greatest advantages of volume sonography is the ability to standardize the examination of volumes, defining spatial relationships between various anatomic planes and organs, and enabling the automatic retrieval of predefined planes of a specific area in question. This has been accomplished by Abuhamad et al. (2004, 2005, 2007) with automation of the fetal heart, and the possible application of the same principles has been addressed in the first-trimester fetus (Abu-Rustum et al. 2012).

PITFALLS IN VOLUME SONOGRAPHY

The basic principle for generating a good 3D image is a good underlying 2D image. For this reason, all the limitations of 2D sonography are manifested in 3D with an added dimension: the quality of the 3D image is limited by the resolution of the 2D image and it becomes critical to optimize the 2D image prior to acquiring a volume in order to obtain the best results. A suboptimal 2D image will result in a suboptimal 3D image. There is a steep learning curve in how to best acquire a 3D volume out of which it is possible to retrieve the optimal images. Resolution is limited in the coronal plane. Although the efficiency of the sonographic machines has improved drastically over the years, volume sonography is more time consuming because considerable time for acquisition and post-processing is still required for optimal results. A good fluid interface is necessary to optimize the image. The third dimension further compounds the introduction of artifacts into the additional dimension, and this is further compounded by the presence of challenging structural anomalies.

The three main factors contributing to artifacts in volume sonography are motion (fetal or maternal), rendering technique (Figure 1.14), and shadowing artifacts (Figure 1.15). Poor rotation and off-center tilt may erroneously be

interpreted as pathology. In addition, artifacts may be a result of manipulation and slicing, such as with the employment of the post-processing tool MagiCut. As such, care must be employed when displaying and interpreting the images.

BASIC CAUSES OF ARTIFACTS

1. Motion of the fetus or mother
2. Rendering techniques
3. Shadowing artifacts

Artifacts may also raise the concern of the family and cause the inexperienced sonographer to overdiagnose (cleft lip) or underdiagnose a certain condition if the area under examination is obscured. In addition, some of the most dangerous artifacts are generated as a result of the use of power and color Doppler. For instance, when evaluating the ventricular septum, erroneous diagnosis of ventricular septal defects may be made.

In gynecology, one of the most significant artifacts is the echo enhancement artifact. This was described by Abuhamad (2006) and is caused by the shadowing in the posterior myometrium, whereby the myometrium now takes on the sonographic appearance of the endometrium. This artifact may occur when attempting to visualize the mid-coronal plane of the uterus, approaching it posterior to the myometrium. If this volume is subsequently rendered in the multiplanar mode, or when obtaining a thick slice, it may be erroneously suggestive of a müllerian abnormality.

CONCLUSION

Volume sonography is here to stay and is of tremendous value in education, consultation, and clarification of challenging findings to both physicians and families. In provides additional information in experienced hands with a properly acquired/displayed volume from an optimally obtained 2D image. Nonetheless, there is a steep learning curve with new terminology and various new technological concepts with which the sonographer must become familiar. In addition, one must keep in mind the inherent limitations, and the sonographer must try to avoid artifacts when acquiring a volume in order to avoid false-positive interpretations and to spare the family undue anxiety.

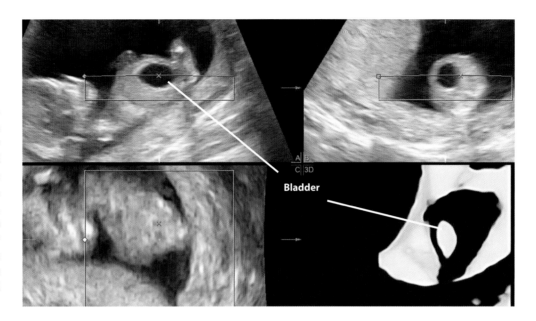

FIGURE 1.10 A 3D volume of a 13w3d fetus where the fetal bladder is clearly visualized in planes A and B. Rendering the volume in the lower right-hand corner, utilizing inversion mode, results in attenuation of the cystic bladder where it now appears echodense, whereas the remaining structures become echolucent, and hence nonvisible.

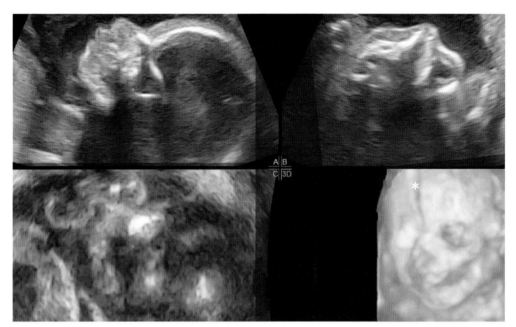

FIGURE 1.11 A 3D rendered volume of a 22w6d fetal face optimized for the maximum mode enabling evaluation of the frontal metopic suture (*).

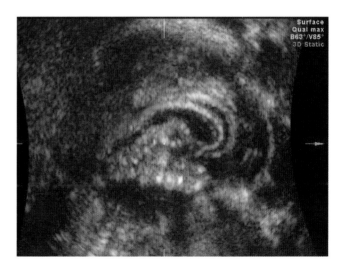

FIGURE 1.12 A 3D volume of a 27w1d fetus from which the mid-coronal plane depicting the corpus callosum was generated. This plane is a challenging plane to obtain by conventional 2D sonography, and with navigation within an optimized volume of the fetal head it becomes feasible

PRACTICAL PEARLS

- Understand the main concepts of volume sonography and the fact that within any volume all the necessary anatomical planes are contained
- Understand the difference between 2D and 3D and the concept of the three orthogonal planes
- Understand the importance of the reference dot as the grounding point in all three planes in the multiplanar mode
- Learn and understand the basic terminology
- Keep in mind both the advantages and the disadvantages of volume sonography
- Be mindful of artifacts and make every attempt to minimize them

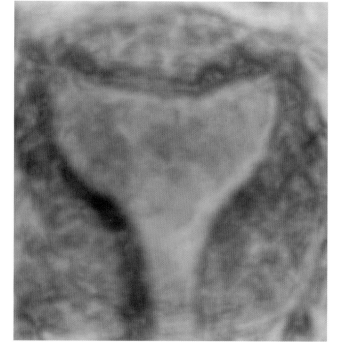

FIGURE 1.13 A transvaginal volume of the uterus during the luteal phase from which the mid-coronal plane is obtained. This allows proper evaluation of the endometrial cavity in order to assess for müllerian abnormalities.

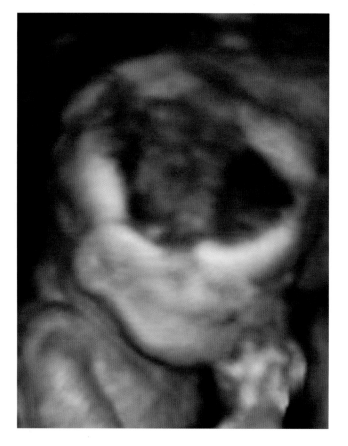

FIGURE 1.14 A 3D surface-rendered volume of a 22w3d fetus. In this volume, rotation of the fetus has generated artifact suggestive of a skull abnormality. Caution must be exercised in such cases to reassure the family as to the well-being of the fetus and to regenerate an artifact-free image of the fetal head.

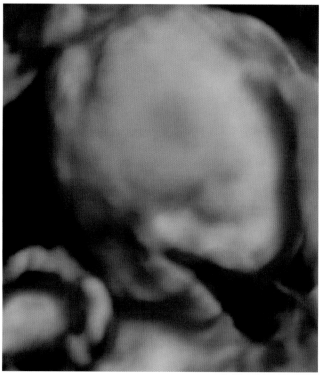

FIGURE 1.15 A 3D surface-rendered volume of a 21w5d fetus using HD*live*. In this volume, shadow artifact by the fetal hand has resulted in an image that may raise concern for a facial cleft. With experience, the sonographer can anticipate such artifacts and would exercise caution prior to generating such images so as to avoid undue parental anxiety.

2 Volume Acquisition

INTRODUCTION

The absolute determining factor for the quality of any 3D/4D volume is the quality of the underlying 2D image and how the actual volume was acquired. As such, one must have the foresight as to what the volume is to be used for so that it is properly acquired in order to be able to generate adequate images for evaluation.

PRINCIPLES OF VOLUME ACQUISITION

Whenever a volume is acquired, there are 3 basic principles to keep in mind for optimization:

1. The target area in question in order to set the size of the box for image acquisition (Figure 2.1)
2. The depth of the structures to be evaluated (angle of acquisition) (Figure 2.2)
3. The quality of the resolution that is desired for optimal image interpretation (quality of acquisition)

Each of the above three prerequisites plays a factor in the time needed to acquire the volume. The greater the requirements, the larger the volume and the higher its resolution, and the more time required to "sweep" through and acquire it, which allows more room for fetal motion and thus artifact introduction. In obstetrical ultrasound, fetal motion becomes a major limiting factor, especially in the B and C planes. For this reason, when fetal motion is anticipated, one must choose the smallest box, the smallest angle, and the least acceptable resolution to swiftly sweep through and acquire as motion-free a volume as possible. In gynecology, and in the absence of any motion of the organs under study, the quality of the volumes acquired is usually not affected by motion. Therefore, the image can be optimized by using a slower sweep speed, thus generating more voxels and a higher-quality image.

VOLUME ACQUISITION

As previously stated, the key to a good 3D volume is an underlying good 2D image and proper acquisition, keeping in mind the three basic keys to acquiring a volume: size of the box, angle of acquisition, and quality of acquisition.

SIZE OF BOX

The size of the box represents the entire area of interest. An example would be when acquiring a volume of the fetal heart at the level of the four-chamber view. The examiner needs to decide how much of the chest is to be included around the heart in order to set the acquisition box around that area of interest. This is exemplified in plane A, the reference plane, in the multiplanar view (Figure 2.1).

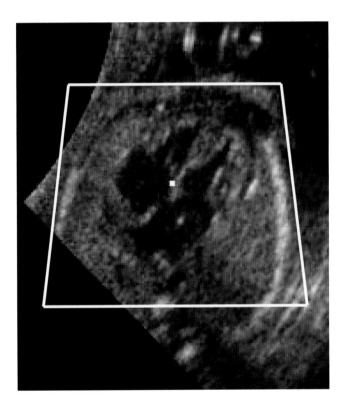

FIGURE 2.1 In order to acquire a 3D volume of the fetal heart at 22w1d, the box of acquisition needs to be placed around the area of interest prior to acquiring the volume. The angle of acquisition is then selected, 30 degrees in this case, and the quality of the volume is selected. The volume is subsequently acquired and saved.

ANGLE OF ACQUISITION

This is determined by how much above and below the area in question the volume should extend. For instance, when acquiring a volume of the fetal heart at the level of the four-chamber view, is the plan to just include the heart or have a volume that spans from the thyroid to the stomach? This is exemplified in plane B, constructed from the 3D volume data set in the multiplanar view (Figure 2.2). The angle depends on the type of transducer being used. In general, it is double the distance that the probe moves on either side of the reference plane. For instance, if the angle chosen is 30 degrees for the fetal heart, then the probe would acquire 15 degrees on either side of (above and below) the four-chamber view, for a total of 30 degrees. Plane C is the third plane, perpendicular to A and B and reconstructed from the volume data set.

QUALITY OF ACQUISITION

The quality of acquisition determines its resolution. The higher the quality, the longer it takes to acquire the volume, thus there is more chance for fetal movement and a greater probability of artifacts. Keep in mind that a higher quality is required for the evaluation of internal structures, whereas a lower quality is sufficient for the evaluation of the external surface. This does not hold true in areas without motion artifact, such as when acquiring a volume of the uterus in gynecology where you can use the widest angle and the largest box with the highest resolution with minimal artifacts generated. Tables 2.1 and 2.2 cover the basic steps for volume acquisition.

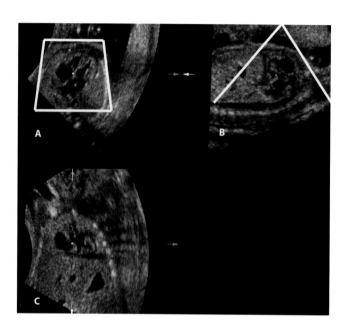

FIGURE 2.2 Once the volume is displayed in the multiplanar mode, plane A depicts the initial 2D plane of acquisition; plane B is perpendicular to it and generally reflects the depth of the structures to be evaluated (angle of acquisition selected for the volume). In this case, 30 degrees is selected, and this includes the area between the stomach all the way cephalad to the thyroid as shown in plane B. plane C is perpendicular to both planes A and B. The quality used for this volume is mid 2. Note that the schematic angle in plane B is not to scale.

Table 2.1 **Steps to Acquiring a Volume of the Fetal Heart and Chest**

Step 1:	Obtain the plane of the four-chamber view after having optimized your basic 2D settings (Figure 2.1)
Step 2:	Select an angle of acquisition of 30 degrees [a]; this volume should subsequently span from the fetal stomach to the thyroid for a second-trimester fetus
Step 3:	Set the quality of the acquisition of the volume to "high" in the absence of fetal motion, and to "medium" in case of fetal motion
Step 4:	Hit "freeze" as this should automatically sweep through the fetal chest, spanning 15 degrees above and below the four-chamber view in order to acquire the volume and display it in the multiplanar mode along the three orthogonal planes
Step 5:	Check plane A to make sure this displays the initially acquired reference plane (Figure 2.2)
Step 6:	Check plane B to make sure it spans from the fetal stomach to the thyroid (Figure 2.2)
Step 7:	Save the volume if it is adequate for later manipulation and offline analysis

[a] The degree of the sweep is related to gestational age. For example, 20 degrees at 20 weeks of gestation, 30 degrees at 30 weeks of gestation.

Table 2.2 **Steps to Acquiring a Volume of the Fetal Face**

Step 1:	Obtain an image of the fetal profile after having optimized your basic 2D settings (Figure 2.3)
Step 2:	Select an angle of acquisition of 65 degrees; this volume should subsequently span the entire width of the fetal face of a second-trimester fetus
Step 3:	Set the quality of the acquisition of the volume to "high" in the absence of fetal motion, and to "medium" in case of fetal motion
Step 4:	Hit "freeze " as this should automatically sweep through the volume, spanning 32.5 degrees on either side of the fetal profile, in order to acquire the volume and display it in the multiplanar mode along the three orthogonal planes
Step 5:	Check plane A to make sure this displays the initially acquired reference plane (Figure 2.4)
Step 6:	Check plane B to make sure it spans the entire width of the fetal face (Figure 2.4)
Step 7:	Save the volume if it is adequate for later manipulation and offline analysis

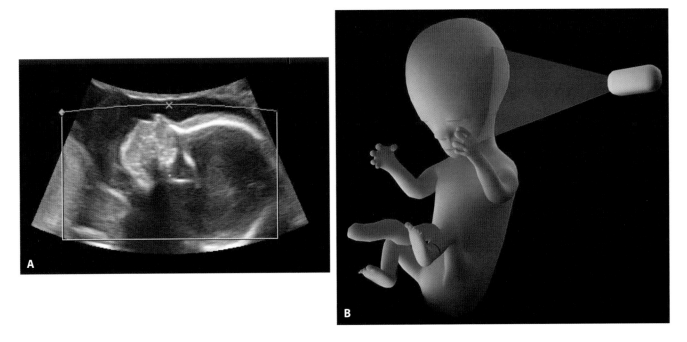

FIGURE 2.3 Face acquisition. (A) In order to acquire a 3D volume of the fetal face, optimize your 2D settings, and place the box of acquisition around the fetal face while attempting to capture the image with a good amniotic fluid interphase in front of the fetal face. The angle of acquisition is then selected, 65 degrees in this example, and the quality of the volume is then set. The volume is subsequently acquired and saved. (B) A 3D model showing the plane of acquisition commencing with the fetal profile.

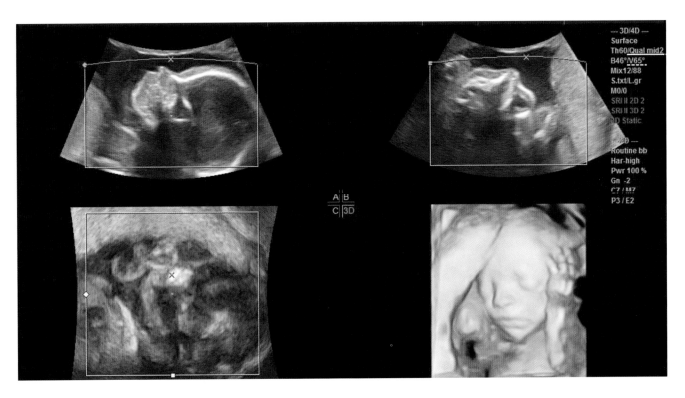

FIGURE 2.4 Once the volume is acquired it may be displayed in the multiplanar mode and surface rendering. Note the position of the box of acquisition in plane A. The depth, represented by the angle of acquisition, is depicted in plane B and encompasses the entire width of the face extending beyond each of the two orbits. The angle of acquisition can be seen in the top right-hand corner (underlined) as mid 2. In addition, the quality of the volume is mid 2 (dashed underline).

CONCLUSION

The key to the success in volume sonography is in an optimal underlying 2D image. The volume should be acquired with the appropriate size with which to fully evaluate the area under examination, keeping in mind the limitations of acquiring a volume of high resolution and a large volume. As a general rule, longer acquisition is accompanied by fetal motion, thus introducing more artifacts.

PRACTICAL PEARLS

- To optimize volume acquisition and to minimize artifact, use the smallest acquisition box, the smallest necessary angle, and the least acceptable quality
- Most sonograghic machines come with factory presets that are helpful whether evaluating the fetal surface, skeleton, or heart, and these presets may be individualized
- Once the ideal settings are arrived at for a particular area, individual settings may be programmed into the system
- For external surfaces, a lower quality may be utilized for volume acquisition
- For internal structures, a higher quality for acquisition yields better results

3 Volume Manipulation

INTRODUCTION

This chapter focuses on volume manipulation so that the user can optimize the image planes for display of the multiplanar (Figure 3.1) and render formats (Figures 3.2 and 3.3).

VOLUME MANIPULATION

After the volume is acquired, it is possible to manipulate and navigate through the volume utilizing the most appropriate technique for a complete assessment of the area of interest. This may be accomplished utilizing rotation through the reference dot along the three axes. The volume may be manipulated further by changing the size and direction from which the region of interest is examined.

BASIC CONCEPTS FOR VOLUME MANIPULATION

1. Placing the reference dot on the target area within the volume
2. Rotating along the *X*, *Y*, and *Z* axes through the reference dot
3. Selecting the size and direction from which to view the region of interest

---

THE REFERENCE DOT

The reference dot is the intersection point between all three orthogonal planes. Volume manipulation is facilitated by placing the reference dot at a specific point within the volume. This subsequently becomes the pivotal point around which the volume may be rotated along any of the three axes, without losing its position, as it remains displayed in all three orthogonal planes. The reference dot can be moved around so that it is set at a particular point of interest within the volume, and it can be seen in all three orthogonal planes simultaneously if the multiplanar mode is selected (Figure 3.4). For instance, if a volume of the fetal abdomen is obtained with the primary focus on the fetal stomach, then the reference dot can be placed on the fetal stomach and it is subsequently identified in all three orthogonal planes (Figure 3.5). In the volume of the fetal abdomen, one would not lose the stomach, if it is the focal point of interest, and any manipulation within that volume will occur around the stomach where it remains clearly displayed at all times and in all three orthogonal or perpendicular planes, as the primary designated structure. If tomographic ultrasound imaging (TUI) were to be utilized, then the reference dot would locate the stomach in each of the planes displayed (Figure 3.6). If the aorta becomes the primary point of interest, then the reference point may be moved from the stomach to the aorta for navigation within the volume, with the aorta as the pivotal point (Figure 3.7).

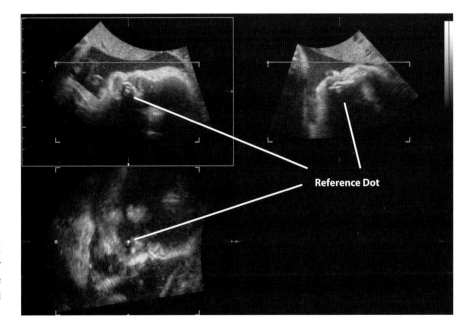

FIGURE 3.1 A 3D volume of the fetal face at 32w1d displayed in the multiplanar mode with the volume displayed in three orthogonal 2D planes – planes A, B, and C – all intersecting in the reference dot.

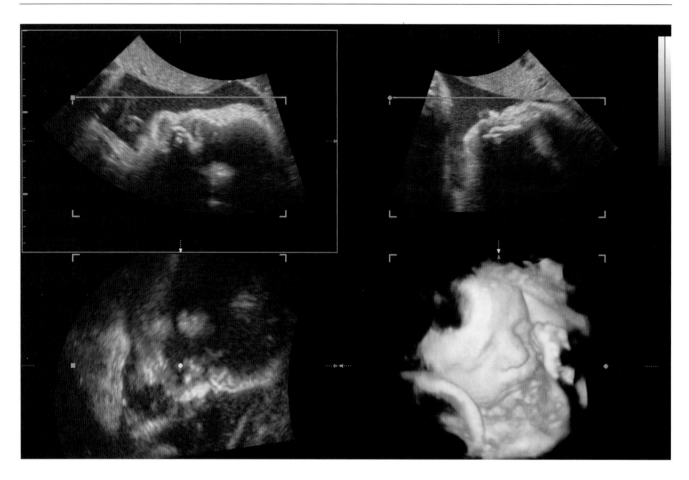

FIGURE 3.2   The same volume from Figure 3.1 displayed using surface rendering. In this case, the sonographer may also select to display the volume in only one pane so that the rendered image will be the only image displayed without showing the images in planes A, B, and C.

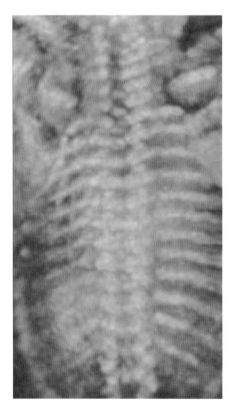

FIGURE 3.3   A 3D volume of a 22w4d fetal chest displayed using the skeleton mode, also known as maximum mode, clearly depicting the rib cage and all 12 ribs. Here the single-pane view has been selected.

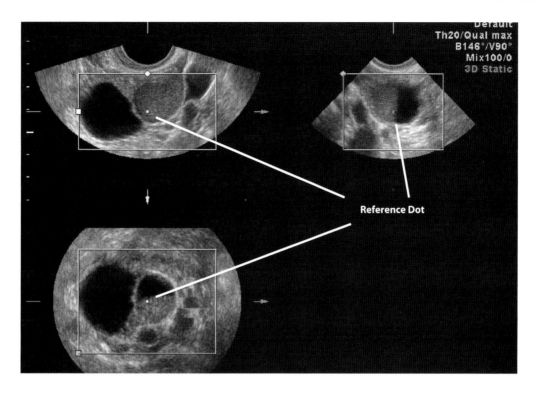

FIGURE 3.4 A transvaginal 3D volume of a multicystic ovary displayed in the three orthogonal planes with the reference dot clearly visible in planes A, B, and C.

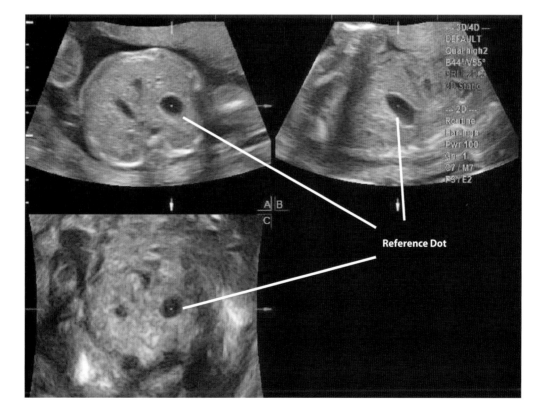

FIGURE 3.5 A 3D volume of the abdomen of a 22w1d fetus acquired with an angle of 55 degrees and a quality of high 2 (information in the top right-hand side of the image) displayed in the multiplanar mode. The reference dot is placed in the fetal stomach, localizing it in each of the three planes.

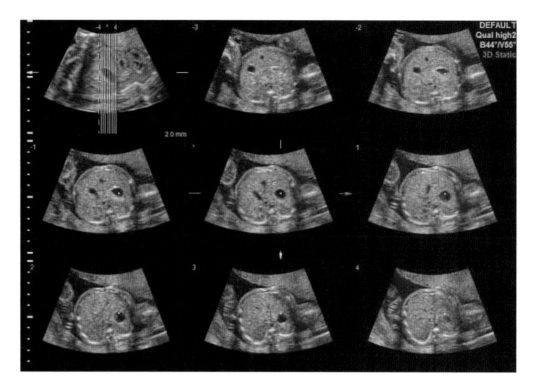

FIGURE 3.6   The same 3D volume obtained for Figure 3.5 is now displayed using TUI with a slice thickness of 2 mm. The reference dot remains in the stomach in all the planes. This becomes most useful in determining spatial relationships between organs, or when evaluating the boundaries of a tumor.

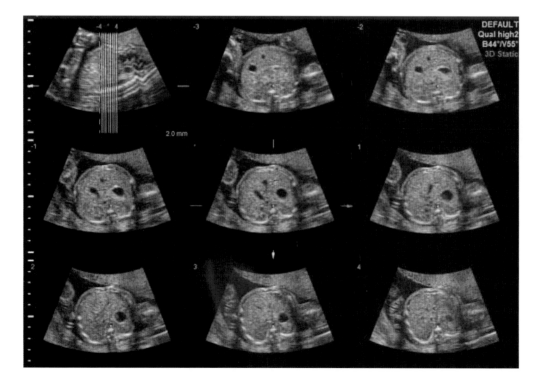

FIGURE 3.7   The same 3D volume obtained for Figures 3.5 and 3.6 is still displayed using TUI with a slice thickness of 2 mm; however, now the reference dot is moved to the aorta and it localizes the aorta in all eight panes.

ROTATION ALONG THE X, Y, AND Z AXES

To further navigate within the volume, rotation can be accomplished along any of the three orthogonal planes (the X, Y, and Z axes), with the reference dot as the point around which the rotation occurs. Rotation along the X axis is accomplished as if rotating in a 'rotisserie' mode (Figure 3.8). Rotation along the Y axis is in the orientation of the motion of a 'drill' (Figure 3.9). Rotation along the Z axis is in a clockwise/counterclockwise fashion within the image through the reference dot, in a 'rocking' motion (Figure 3.10).

SCROLLING THROUGH THE VOLUME

It is also possible to scroll through the volume moving cephalad or caudad. This can be carried out in any of the three orthogonal planes. For example, in the volume of a first-trimester fetus, this may be accomplished by moving the reference dot in plane A cephalad to reach the fetal head in plane B (Figure 3.11), or caudad to reach the fetal abdomen in plane B (Figure 3.12). This may also be accomplished using the 'depth' button on the machine.

BASIC CONCEPTS IN ROTATING AROUND AN AXIS THROUGH THE REFERENCE DOT

1. X axis rotation is similar to the motion of a 'rotisserie'
2. Y axis rotation is similar to the motion of a 'drill'
3. Z axis rotation is similar to a back and forth 'rocking' motion

---

BASIC CONCEPTS FOR SCROLLING THROUGH THE VOLUME

1. Scrolling may be accomplished by moving the reference dot
2. Scrolling may be accomplished by using the 'depth' button

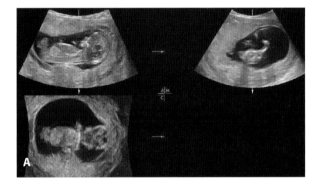
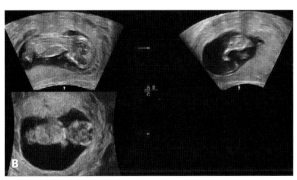
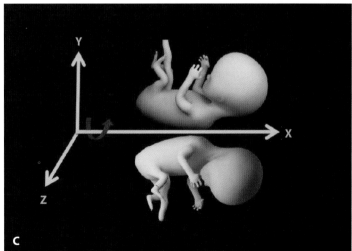

FIGURE 3.8 3D volume of a 12w6d fetus displayed in the multiplanar mode. (A) The initial volume. (B) The volume after it has been rotated along the X axis through the reference dot in the fetal neck in reference plane A as if rotated around a rotisserie. (C) 3D model depicting X rotation.

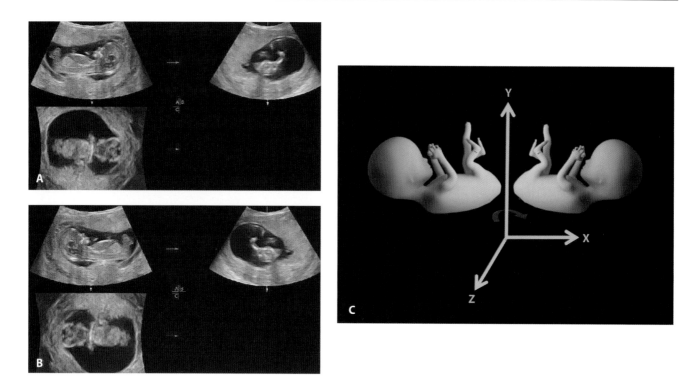

FIGURE 3.9   3D volume of a 12w6d fetus displayed in the multiplanar mode. (A) Initial volume. (B) Volume after it has been rotated along the *Y* axis through the reference dot in the fetal neck in reference plane A as if rotated along the rotational axis of a drill. (C) 3D model depicting *Y* rotation.

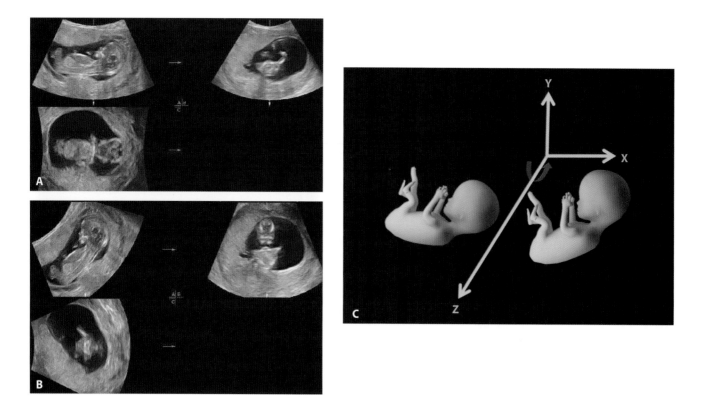

FIGURE 3.10   3D volume of a 12w6d fetus displayed in the multiplanar mode. (A) Initial volume. (B) Volume after it has been rotated along the *Z* axis through the reference dot in the fetal neck in reference plane A as if in a rocking motion. (C) 3D model depicting *Z* rotation.

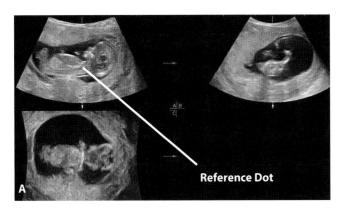

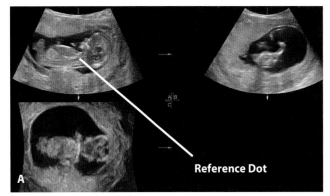

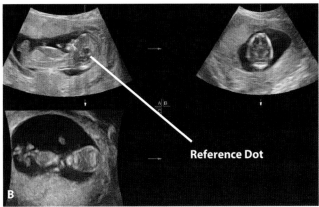

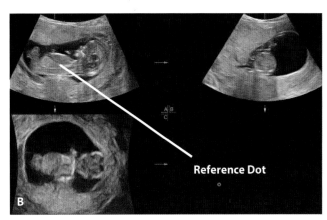

FIGURE 3.11 3D volume of a 12w6d fetus displayed in the multiplanar mode. (A) Initial volume with the reference dot at the level of the fetal neck in plane A generating an axial image of the neck in plane B. (B) Volume after the reference dot in plane A has been moved cephalad to the fetal head generating a new image in plane B of the fetal cranium.

FIGURE 3.12 3D volume of a 12w6d fetus displayed in the multiplanar mode. (A) Initial volume with the reference dot at the level of the fetal neck in plane A generating an axial image of the neck in plane B. (B) Volume after the reference dot in plane A has been moved caudad to the fetal abdomen generating a new image in plane B of the fetal abdominal circumference plane with a visible fetal stomach.

SIZE AND DIRECTION OF THE REGION OF INTEREST

Another way to manipulate the volume, in the render mode, is by changing the direction and/or size with which the region of interest is viewed. For any volume displayed in the three orthogonal planes in the multiplanar mode, the reference plane is plane A. With the acquisition box still visible in plane A, it is clear that it has four sides (Figure 3.13). Any of these four sides may then be selected as the direction from which to view the volume or render it. In addition, the size

of the acquisition box may be changed to focus on a specific area outside or within the volume. For instance, the same volume may be viewed from the top down (Figure 3.14) or from the bottom up (Figure 3.15). This is depicted by the green color, signaling the direction of viewing the region of interest (Figures 3.14 and 3.15). The size of the box may also be altered to look within the volume – for example, to evaluate the fetal stomach in a volume of the fetal abdomen (Figure 3.16).

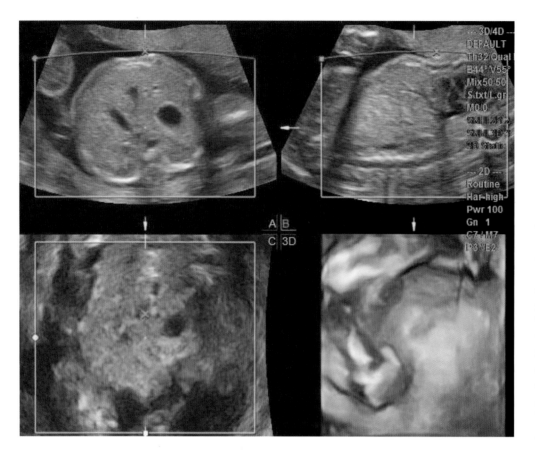

FIGURE 3.13 3D volume of the fetal abdomen of a 22w1d fetus. Note the box of acquisition. It has four sides. The green side indicates the direction of viewing the region of interest. The sides of the box indicate the borders of the region of interest which is large in this example. In this volume, the direction of viewing/rendering the volume is top to bottom, as indicated by the green line.

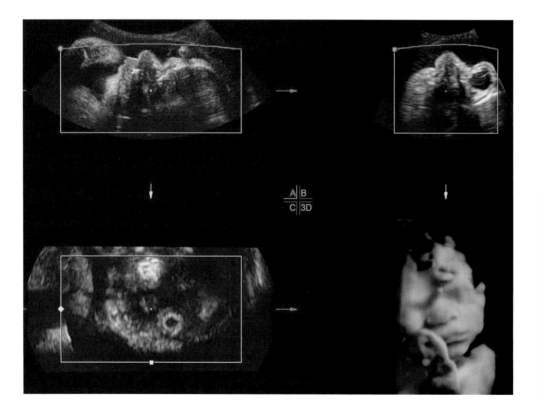

FIGURE 3.14 3D volume of a 32w5d fetal face displayed in the multiplanar mode and surface rendered using HD*live*. The direction of evaluating/rendering the region of interest is top to bottom as indicated by the green line in plane A, enabling visualization of the fetal face. The umbilical cord creates an artifact along the forehead.

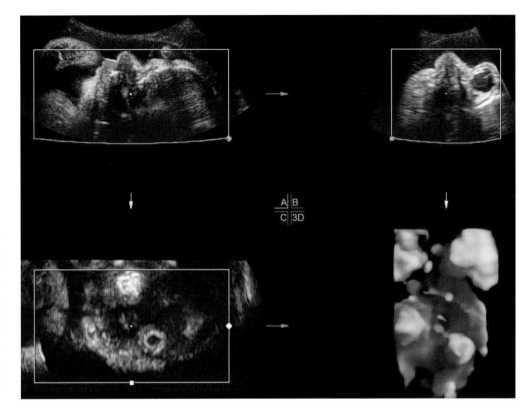

FIGURE 3.15 This is the same volume rendered in Figure 3.14; however, in this instance the direction of the region of interest is flipped 180 degrees. It is bottom to top, as indicated by the line in plane A. As a consequence, the final rendered image is not clear and does not depict the fetal face.

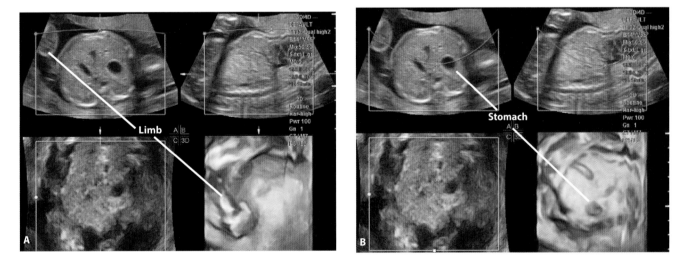

FIGURE 3.16 This is the same 3D volume of Figure 3.13. (A) The region of interest encompasses the entire abdomen with the direction of view top to bottom starting outside the fetal skin as depicted by the line in plane A. This is depicted in the final rendered image where a fetal limb is seen. (B) The size of the region of interest is changed and now the green viewing line starts at the level of the fetal stomach, which can be seen in the final rendered image.

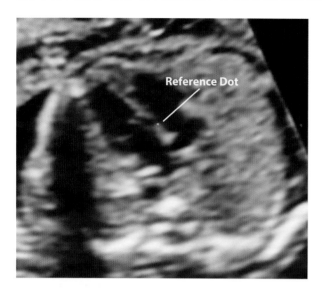

FIGURE 3.17 3D volume of the heart of a 21w6d fetus is acquired and displayed in a single-pane view from plane A, with the reference dot placed along the crux of the heart.

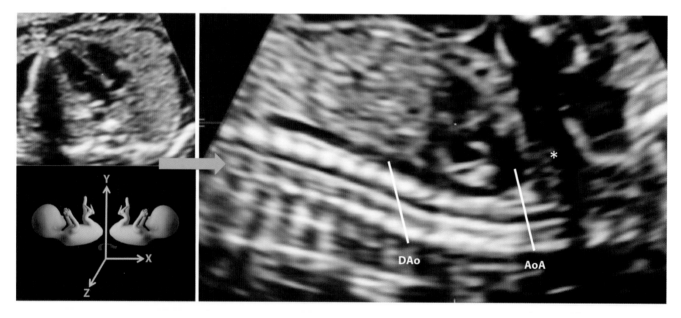

FIGURE 3.18 This is the same volume as in Figure 3.17. "Spinning" along the *Y* axis is carried out, resulting in complete visualization of the aortic arch (AoA), head and neck vessels (*), and the descending aorta (DAo)

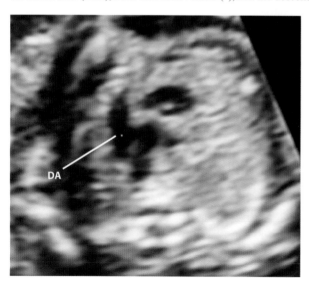

FIGURE 3.19 Scrolling cephalad from the four-chamber view in Figure 3.17, the three-vessel view is generated with the reference dot placed along the ductus arteriosus (DA).

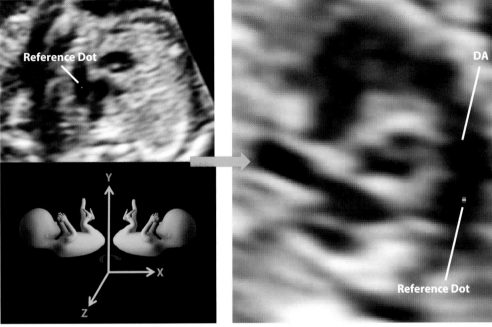

FIGURE 3.20 Commencing from the image in Figure 3.19, where the reference dot was placed in the ductus arteriosus, it is possible to "spin" along the Y axis in order to generate a view of the ductus arteriosus (DA).

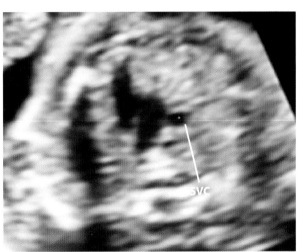

FIGURE 3.21 Returning to the three-vessel view, the reference dot is now placed along the superior vena cava (SVC).

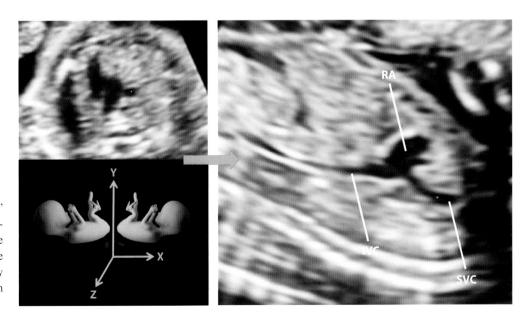

FIGURE 3.22 "Spinning" along the Y axis now generates the bicaval view with the superior and inferior venae cavae (SVC, IVC) clearly seen entering the right atrium (RA).

DEVORE'S SPIN TECHNIQUE

The perfect example to illustrate the rotation along the three axes along a fixed reference point is DeVore's spin technique for evaluating the fetal heart (DeVore et al. 2004). Table 3.1 describes, in a stepwise fashion, how rotation along the X and Y axes and navigating through a volume acquired at the level of the four-chamber views allows the display of the outflow tracts.

Table 3.1 **Steps in the Spin Technique Displaying the Outflow Tracts Out of a Volume of the Fetal Chest**

Step 1:	Select the 4 chamber view as your reference plane with the ultrasound beam perpendicular to the ventricular septum (Figure 3.17)
Step 2:	Obtain a 3D sweep with an angle of acquisition of 30 degrees and a mid to high quality for the volume
Step 4:	Place the reference point along the crux of the heart (Figure 3.17)
Step 5:	Rotate the volume along the Y axis to depict the aortic arch along its entire length (Figure 3.18)
Step 6:	Go back to the initial volume and scroll cephalad to the 3-vessel view and place the reference dot on the ductus arteriosus (Figure 3.19)
Step 7:	Rotate along the Y axis to depict the ductal arch (Figure 3.20)
Step 8:	Go back to the 3-vessel view and place the reference dot in the superior vena cava (Figure 3.21)
Step 9:	Rotate along the Y axis to depict the bicaval view with the superior and inferior venae cavae visible entering the right atrium (Figure 3.22)

CONCLUSION

A volume may be manipulated by rotation along the X, Y, and Z axes, with the reference dot serving as the pivotal point around which the rotation is carried out. In addition, it is possible to scroll through any volume, along any of the three planes, by moving the reference dot or by utilizing the "depth" button available on the ultrasound machines. Adjusting the size of the region of interest and the direction of viewing enables the external or in-depth study of any volume. The sonographer's clear understanding of how to manipulate the acquired volume, coupled with the knowledge of which rendering technique is optimal for each particular area under study, is critical to enable the varied and detailed study of the developing fetus, as illustrated in subsequent chapters.

PRACTICAL PEARLS

- The reference dot is the pivotal point around which to navigate through the volume
- Remember the three main analogies of rotating around the three axes: rotisserie (X), drill (Y), and rocking (Z) (Abuhamad oral communication 2004)
- You may scroll through the volume utilizing parallel shift or by moving the reference dot
- Whenever a volume is displayed in the multiplanar mode, any of the three planes A, B, or C may be selected for further manipulation. The activated image/plane is designated by a scale next to it
- Any volume may be viewed from four directions, represented by the four sides of the acquisition box in reference plane A or whichever of the three planes is selected as the reference plane

4 Volume Display

INTRODUCTION

Once a 3D volume is acquired, it may be displayed in the multiplanar mode, discussed in Chapter 3, or it may be rendered in a multitude of other ways, the most recognized of which is the surface mode (Figure 4.1), depicting the fetal face. The surface mode is the most commonly used display mode to demonstrate features of the fetal face. Unfortunately, this display format has generated a bad name for 3D ultrasound because of its nonmedical use for "entertainment ultrasound." This becomes more problematic with the advent of HD*live* (Figure 4.2) and the amazingly lifelike quality of the fetal images. Although 3D ultrasound may sometimes be misused, it has tremendous potential as a diagnostic tool to assist the clinician and sonographer in the quest for detailed evaluation of anatomical structures.

There are various additional rendering modalities with which to display a volume such as the maximum mode (for display of the skeleton) and minimum and inversion modes (for display of vascular and fluid-filled structures). To complement the various display modes, different rendering colors can be selected to optimize the visualization of the target area in question. These may be combined in a multitude of ways, and this is the focus of this chapter.

When rendering a volume, manipulation along the three axes may still be required for image optimization. In addition, the orientation from which to view the acquired volume may be altered by changing the direction of the region of interest (ROI). This allows for viewing a specific area from any of the four sides. An example would be looking at the atrioventricular (AV) valves. The approach may be from the apical or the basal orientation (Figure 4.3 and 4.4). Table 4.1 covers a stepwise approach to altering the ROI orientation in order to visualize the AV valves.

For the various rendering modes, the 2D image settings must be optimized and a sweep through the area in question is obtained, and subsequently the various rendering modalities may be utilized.

SURFACE RENDERING/HD*live*

In surface rendering of the fetal face, a prerequisite is a good fluid interphase in front of the fetal face. In addition, one must acquire a volume without the fetal cord or extremities covering the face, and at a time when there is minimal fetal motion. In order to obtain a 3D image of the fetal profile, the volume must also be acquired en face (Figure 4.5). If the goal is to obtain a portrait of the fetal face, the volume acquisition begins by imaging the fetal profile (Figure 4.6). The volume may be obtained using either of the above approaches and manipulated to generate the face or profile. However, this approach may result in the introduction of additional artifacts, hindering the quality of the final rendered images.

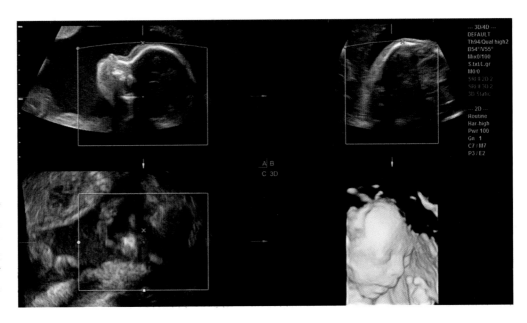

FIGURE 4.1 A 3D volume of a 23w4d fetal face displayed in the multiplanar mode and rendered using surface rendering. Note the size of the box for the region of interest, the direction of viewing the region of interest (top to bottom), the quality of the acquired volume (set at high 2) and the angle of acquisition of 55 degrees (top right-hand corner).

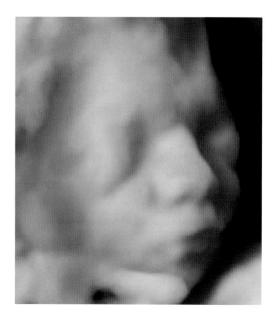

FIGURE 4.2 A 3D volume of the fetal face at 21w6d displayed using HD*live*, a new surface-rendering mode with an adjustable internal light source.

Table 4.1 **Steps in Altering the ROI Orientation while Viewing the AV Valves**

Step 1:	Select the four-chamber view as your reference plane with the ultrasound beam parallel to the ventricular septum
Step 2:	Obtain a 3D sweep with an angle of acquisition of 15 degrees and a mid to high quality for the volume
Step 3:	Place the render box over the AV valves with the ROI orientation from the basal (atrial) side
Step 4:	The AV valves are now depicted in the rendered image (Figure 4.3)
Step 5:	Change the ROI orientation now to the apical (ventricular side) (Figure 4.4)
Step 6:	The leaflets of the AV valves may now be visualized from the ventricular side in the final rendered image

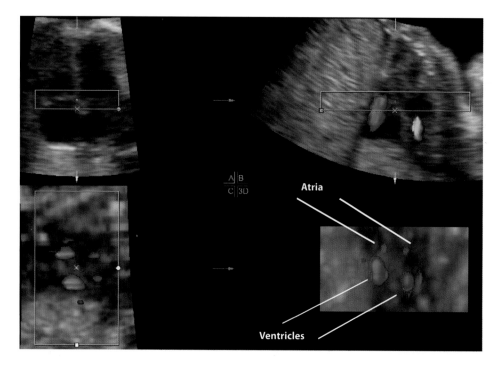

FIGURE 4.3 A 3D volume with color Doppler of the heart of a 25w4d fetus displayed using the glass body mode which minimizes the gray scale and highlights the color Doppler. Here the box for the region of interest has been set to include the atrioventricular valves with a direction from bottom to top, basal approach, depicting looking down from the atria. Note the closed valves during systole.

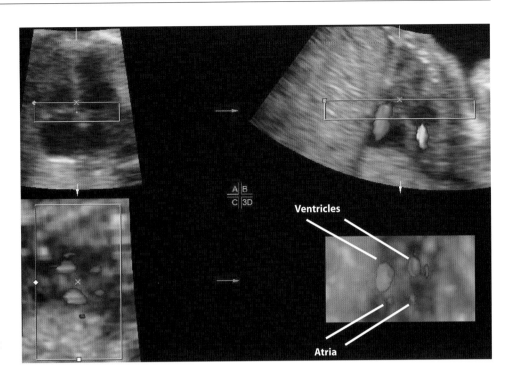

FIGURE 4.4 The same 3D volume with color Doppler of the heart of a 25w4d fetus from figure 4.3 displayed using the the glass body mode, which minimizes the gray scale and highlights the color Doppler. Again, the box for the region of interest has been set to include the atrioventricular valves; however in this case, the direction of view is from top to bottom, apical view, depicting looking up from the ventricles. Note the closed valves during systole.

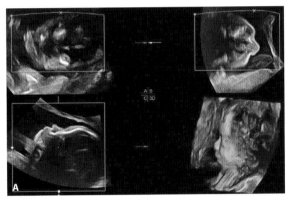
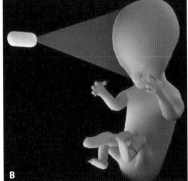

FIGURE 4.5 Acquisition for generating the fetal profile. (A) A 3D volume of the fetal face of a 26w1d fetus. In order to depict the fetal profile, the acquisition plane A must be en face with a good amniotic fluid interphase in front of the fetal face. Note the size of the region of interest and the direction of view being top to bottom. (B) A 3D model depicting an en face acquisition.

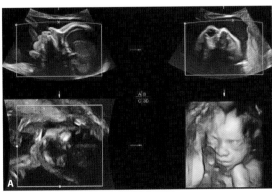
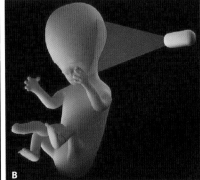

FIGURE 4.6 Acquisition for visualizing the fetus en face. (A) A 3D volume of the fetal face of a 26w1d fetus, the same fetus in figure 4.5. However, in this case, In order to depict the fetal face en face, the acquisition plane (A) must be of the fetal profile with a good amniotic fluid interphase in front of the fetal face. Note the size of the region of interest and the direction of view being top to bottom. (B) A 3D model depicting a side acquisition.

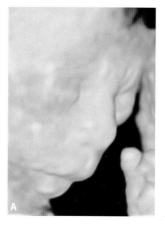 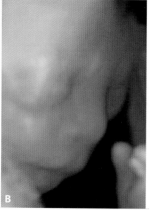 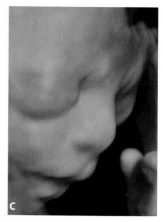

FIGURE 4.7 A 3D volume of the face of a 23w4d fetus rendered using various modalities. (A) Surface rendering using default settings. (B) Dynamic rendering. (C) *HDlive.*

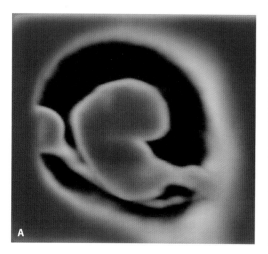 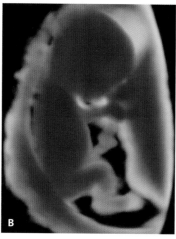

FIGURE 4.8 A transvaginal 3D volume of an (A) 8w0d fetus, (B) 12w4d fetus fetus surface rendered using HD*live*. However, in this case, the light source was moved so that it shone from behind the fetus creating these unique image.

The rendered image may be displayed in the surface mode (default setting on most machines); dynamic rendering; or HD*live* (Figure 4.7), which utilizes sophisticated skin-rendering techniques to generate lifelike images. The sonographer must keep in mind that for optimal results, it is necessary to remove any cord, placenta, or extremities by the electronic scalpel (MagiCut) and to optimize the image prior to activating HD*live*. A unique feature of HD*live* is the availability of a movable internal light source that may be adjusted for optimal image display (Figure 4.8).

**BASIC CONCEPTS IN OBTAINING
A SURFACE-RENDERED IMAGE
OF THE FETAL FACE**

1. A fluid–tissue interphase is required for optimal rendering of the image
2. Avoid obtaining a volume with the fetal cord or an extremity covering the face
3. To visualize the fetus face en face, start with the fetal profile (sagittal view) as the reference plane
4. To visualize the fetal profile, start with an en face reference plane (coronal view) of the fetal face

---

MAXIMUM MODE

The maximum mode is utilized to display the fetal skeleton – the ribs, spine, extremities, bony face, sutures of the fetal skull, or cranium. The same basic principles of volume acquisition discussed in Chapter 2 apply here with respect to volume acquisition and the need to optimize the basic 2D image. However, when choosing the "render" mode, the maximum mode is selected and the region of interest is selected around the area in question (Figure 4.9).

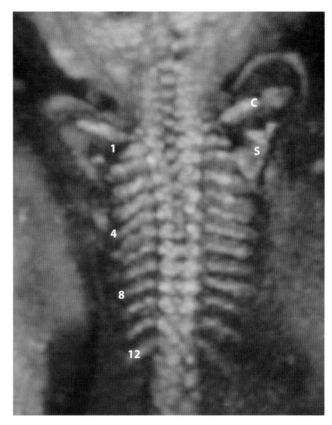

FIGURE 4.9 A 3D volume of a 21w4d fetus displayed in the skeletal (maximum) mode. Note that this mode highlights the bony structures and enables visualizing the clavicles (C), scapula (S) as well as all 12 ribs (1–12).

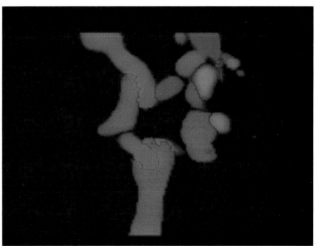

FIGURE 4.10 A 3D volume of the Circle of Willis with color Doppler in a 22w36d fetus displayed using the minimum mode, which removes all gray scale.

MINIMUM MODE/GLASS BODY MODE

Whenever vascular or fluid-filled structures such as fetal vessels, heart, stomach, kidneys, or bladder are under examination, the minimum mode may be utilized. The minimum mode optimizes the parameters for visualizing the *echolucent* areas. For example, if the Circle of Willis is to be evaluated, the 2D and color Doppler image settings should be optimized and the Circle of Willis should be the starting reference plane when acquiring the volume. A 3D sweep may then be obtained, and the minimum mode is selected in order to remove all the gray-scale areas and to highlight the vasculature of the Circle of Willis, where color Doppler is also employed (Figure 4.10). In addition, high-definition flow and B flow may be utilized instead of color Doppler to further evaluate the area under study. The glass body mode is a compromise between minimum mode and regular imaging, where the gray scale is minimized but not completely removed. This aids in maintaining the volume orientation of the vasculature within the anatomical structures being studied (Figure 4.11).

INVERSION MODE

The inversion mode is usually complementary to the minimum mode, where the echolucent area under study in the minimum mode may be "inverted" so that the gray scale is minimized and echolucent structures become echogenic, further facilitating characterization and volume calculation of the area in question. An example of the utility of the inversion mode is in evaluating a multicystic ovary (Figure 4.12). In addition, the inversion mode is useful for rendering a cast of the area in question; for instance a ventricular septal defect (VSD) (Figure 4.13). A stepwise approach to inverting a volume is described in Table 4.2.

Table 4.2 **Steps for Employing Inversion Mode in a Cystic Ovary**

Step 1:	Acquire a volume of the adnexa and display it in the multiplanar mode using maximal quality (Figure 4.12a)
Step 2:	Select the inversion mode and render the volume (Figure 4.12b)
Step 3:	Change the direction of the region of interest as needed (Figure 4.12c)
Step 4:	Utilize MagiCut and adjust the threshold, transparency, and color of the image for optimal results (Figure 4.12c)

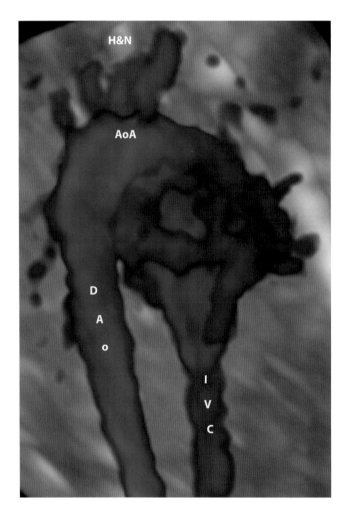

FIGURE 4.11 A sagittal 3D volume of a 22w6d fetus with color Doppler displayed using glass body mode. Here the gray scale is minimized and the fetal vasculature is highlighted. In this case, the aortic arch (AoA), with the head and neck vessels (H & N), descending aorta (DAo) as well as the inferior vena cava (IVC) are seen.

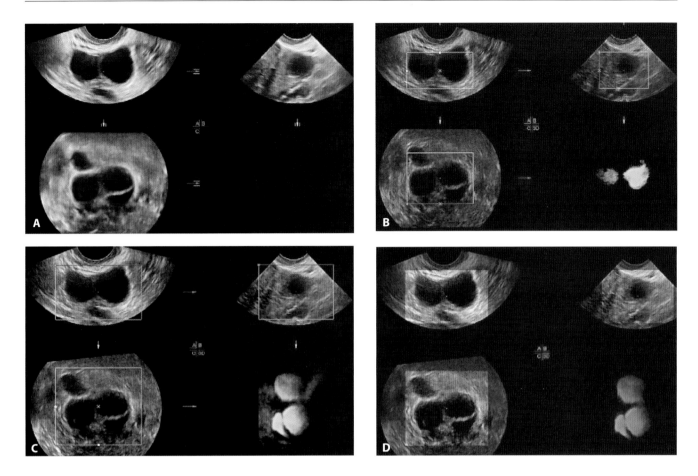

FIGURE 4.12 A transvaginal 3D volume of a multicystic ovary rendered using inversion mode. (A) Multiplanar display using VCI at a slice thickness of 2 mm. (B) The volume is rendered using inversion mode. (C) The direction of the region of interest is changed to "top to bottom" in reference plane A. (D) MagiCut as well as manipulation of the threshold, transparency and color are carried out for optimal results for visualizing the cysts.

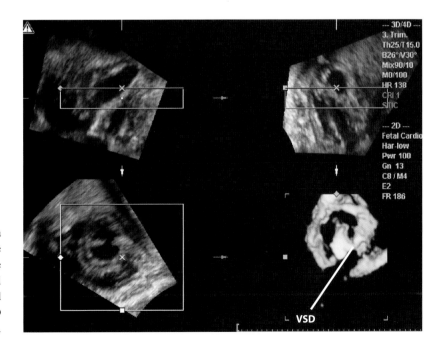

FIGURE 4.13 A 3D volume of the heart of a 32w0d fetus displayed in the multiplanar mode with rendering using the inversion mode. The fetus was found to have a ventricular septal defect (VSD) whose presence was confirmed using inversion mode. The flow across the VSD is now highlighted as seen in the rendered image.

TOMOGRAPHIC ULTRASOUND IMAGING (TUI)

Tomographic ultrasound imaging (TUI) is the sonographic equivalent of CT scanning. Utilizing this volume mode enables the generation of multiple slices of the acquired volume under study, to a set distance in mm, in any of the three orthogonal planes, in a chosen number of panes. This is of particular utility in the first trimester, where a single volume can be obtained of the entire fetus and then, utilizing TUI, most of the fetal anatomic and biometric planes may be generated, starting from the transverse plane of the abdominal circumference (Figure 4.14). TUI is also of utmost utility in determining the size of a mass or lesion and its relationship to the adjacent organs. It facilitates mapping the lesion's locale to within 0.5 mm and aids in determining the extent of spread to and involvement of surrounding structures.

CONCLUSION

The trilogy of volume acquisition, manipulation, and display form the foundation for optimal image generation when employing 3D ultrasound. The sonographer must become familiar with all the key components and must not be afraid to experiment with the various modalities in order to gain expertise and maximize the use of the various capabilities of the sonographic machine.

PRACTICAL PEARLS

- There are several rendering modalities that may be utilized depending on the area under study
- The minimum mode is ideal for fluid-filled structures such as the heart and vessels
- The maximum mode is ideal for evaluating the bony structures
- Optimization of the underlying 2D image prior to volume acquisition is critical
- Rotation along the three axes as well as scrolling within the volume further refine the quality of the rendered image
- Though one is tempted to immediately utilize HD*live* for the evaluation of the fetal face, a higher-quality image is generated if the volume is first acquired using the default settings; once the image gain and threshold have been adjusted and MagiCut utilized, HD*live* may be activated for optimal results (Benoit, oral communication 2012)

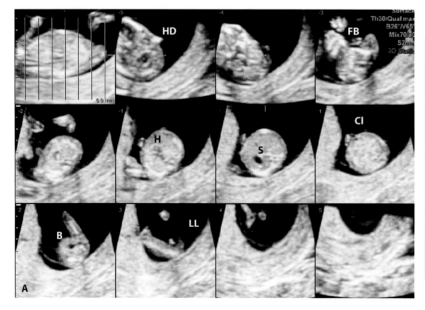
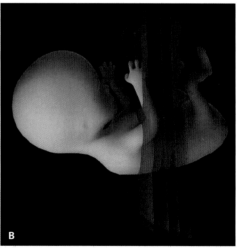

FIGURE 4.14 Tomographic ultrasound imaging (TUI). (A) A 3D volume of a 12w5d fetus displayed using TUI with an interslice distance of 6 mm and VCI at a slice thickness of 2 mm. The planes depicting the head (HD), facial bones (FB), heart (H), stomach (S), cord insertion (CI), bladder (B), and lower limbs (LL) are generated out of the volume. (B) A 3D model depicting the axial slicing of TUI.

5 Spatiotemporal Image Correlation

INTRODUCTION

Spatiotemporal image correlation (STIC) was first introduced by DeVore et al. in 2003 (DeVore et al. 2003; Viñals et al. 2003). It is a unique volume sonographic feature in which a 4D volume of the fetal heart is acquired. Acquiring the volume using STIC overlays multiple 2D images of the beating heart, generating a volume of a full cardiac cycle that may then be displayed as 2D images (Figure 5.1) or a continuous cineloop. It is considered a 4D technique because the volume is displayed in motion, and various color modalities may be incorporated into the volume as well (Figure 5.2). In addition, this volume of the beating heart may be manipulated along any of the 3D orthogonal planes and through any selected reference point, and may be studied while beating through a full cardiac cycle. Combining a STIC volume with TUI provides invaluable information as well where the image resolution may be enhanced by activating VCI.

SPATIOTEMPORAL IMAGE CORRELATION (STIC)

STIC has had well-documented utility in the evaluation of the fetal heart throughout gestation. There is ample literature explaining the technology (DeVore et al. 2003; Viñals et al. 2003; Chaoui et al. 2004) and addressing its use in the study of normal anatomy and standardizing the approach to the evaluation of the various cardiac planes (Paladini et al. 2008b; Rizzo et al. 2008; Yeo and Romero 2013), in the study of cardiac function (Molina et al. 2008; Uittenbogaard et al. 2009; Hamill et al. 2011; Simioni et al. 2011), and in the evaluation of congenital heart defects (Viñals et al. 2006; Gindes et al. 2009; Turan et al. 2014). In addition, STIC has enabled the off-line consultation with experts for the analysis of stored STIC volumes, which allows the expert to evaluate the fetal heart in a full cardiac cycle at a remote site (Espinoza et al. 2010).

BASIC CONCEPTS IN OBTAINING A STIC VOLUME

1. An apical view for acquisition is ideal
2. Avoid obtaining a volume with an extremity in front of the chest
3. When setting the acquisition box, include the fetal heart and not the entire chest
4. The angle of acquisition need not be more than 15 to 20 degrees

---

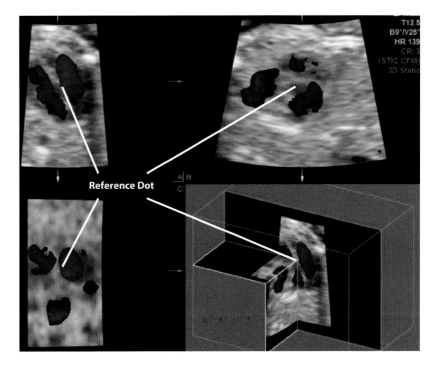

FIGURE 5.1 A 4D STIC volume of a 21w3d fetus acquired with color Doppler at an angle of 25 degrees. It is displayed in the multiplanar "niche" mode. The image in the bottom right-hand corner locates precisely where we are within the volume, with the reference dot as the pivotal point clearly displayed in all four panes.

The uniqueness of this technique is that the fetal heart can be examined off-line, throughout a full cardiac cycle, during systole (Figure 5.3) and diastole (Figure 5.4), allowing a complete and thorough evaluation of both structure and function. Navigating through a STIC volume enables the study of wall motion (the study of atrioventricular and semilunar valves in systole and diastole) (Figures 5.5 and 5.6). Certain manufacturers have made it possible to carry out the off-line M-mode analysis on a STIC volume, and it is possible to change the orientation of the M-line (Figure 5.7). It is also possible to invert a STIC volume (Figure 5.8) and to add it to any of the color modes—color Doppler, power Doppler, or high-definition flow – to further study the valves and the vasculature in motion.

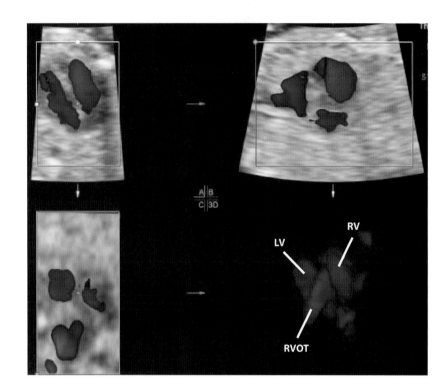

FIGURE 5.2 The same STIC volume from Figure 5.1 rendered using minimum mode, in a back-to-front direction in plane B, depicting the right ventricle (RV) and left ventricle (LV) as well as the right ventricular outflow tract (RVOT).

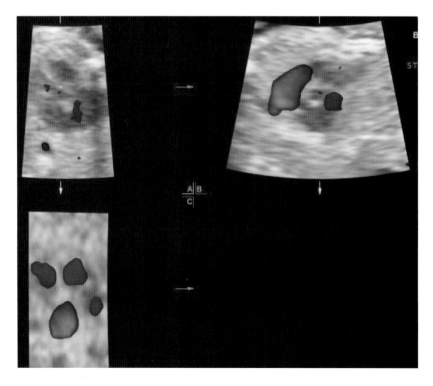

FIGURE 5.3 Navigating through the same STIC volume enables evaluation of the beating heart throughout the cardiac cycle in all three planes simultaneously. This depiction is during systole, with the atrioventricular valves closed and the ventricles empty.

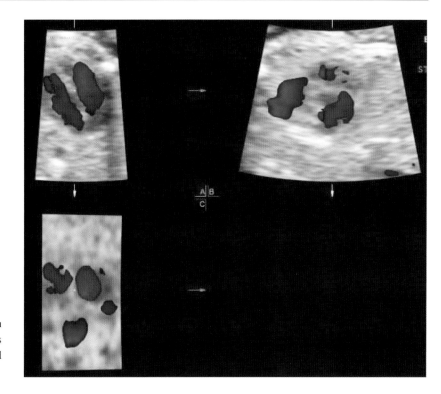

FIGURE 5.4 The same STIC volume with color Doppler in diastole, with good flow across the atrioventricular valves and symmetrical and equal filling of both ventricles.

FIGURE 5.5 The same STIC volume displayed in the three orthogonal planes, with the reference dot in the left ventricular outflow tract. (A) Systole with the aortic valve (AV) open and with complete disappearance of the leaflets of the AV as localized by the reference dot. (B) Diastole with the AV closed and the leaflets visible as an echogenic bright center, as localized by the reference dot.

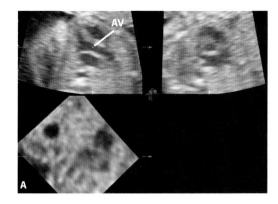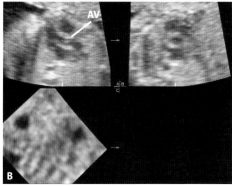

FIGURE 5.6 The same STIC volume displayed in the three orthogonal planes with the reference dot in the right ventricular outflow tract. (A) Systole with the pulmonic valve (PV) open and with complete disappearance of the leaflets of the PV as localized by the reference dot. (B) Diastole with the PV closed and the leaflets visible, as localized by the reference dot.

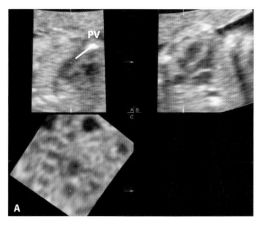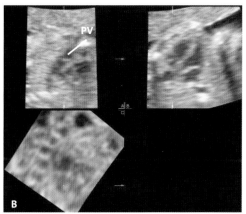

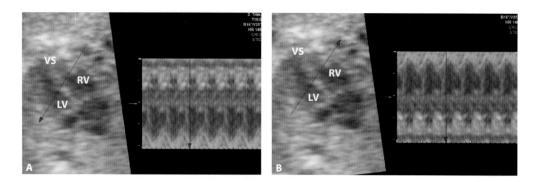

FIGURE 5.7 The same STIC volume displayed using M-mode. (A) Orientation for the M-mode display starts with the right ventricle (RV), the ventricular septum (VS), then the left ventricle (LV). (B) M-line is rotated off-line 180 degrees, whereby the orientation for the M-mode display now becomes reversed starting with the LV, VS, then RV.

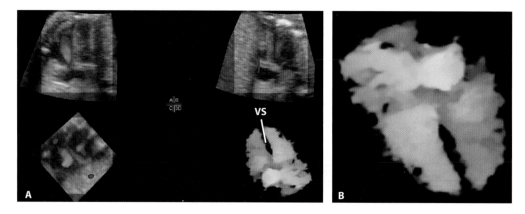

FIGURE 5.8 A STIC volume of a 25w4d fetal heart rendered using inversion mode. (A) Multiplanar display with render using inversion mode. (B) Single pane displayed of a rotated final-rendered volume. This generates a cast of the heart showing the shape of the atria, the ventricles, and the symmetry. Note the intact ventricular septum (VS). When the cineloop is activated the function may also be assessed.

A main limitation of this technique is the resolution in the B and C planes (Figures 5.1, 5.2, 5.5, and 5.6). If the ultimate goal is the sagittal examination of the aortic and sagittal arches or the right atrial inflow, the volume should be acquired in the sagittal plane and not constructed from the four-chamber view, because the reconstruction would result in much loss of resolution. In addition, TUI may be employed to retrieve all the respective anatomical planes out of the volume (Figure 5.9) (DeVore et al. 2004). Table 5.1 covers the basic steps for inverting a STIC volume of the fetal heart, which may be visualized in a multitude of ways, including a 3D cineloop (Figures 5.10–5.15).

Table 5.1 **Steps to Obtaining and Inverting a STIC of the Fetal Heart**

Step 1:	Select the four-chamber view as your reference plane with the ultrasound beam parallel to the ventricular septum
Step 2:	Obtain a 4D sweep with the acquisition box placed just around the heart, with an angle of acquisition of 15 to 30 degrees and a mid to high quality for the volume
Step 3:	Acquire the volume with color Doppler; the STIC volume is now displayed in the multiplanar mode in the three orthogonal planes as cineloops of the beating heart (Figure 5.10)
Step 4:	Render the volume with the direction of the region of interest as a back-to-front direction (Figure 5.11)
Step 5:	Select inversion mode to invert the STIC volume and obtain a 4D inverted cast of the fetal heart; with the current settings, there will be no clear cast (Figure 5.12)
Step 6:	Adjust the threshold to roughly 120 and the mix to 100/0 to optimize the final rendered image (Figure 5.13)
Step 7:	Select the single-image mode and rotate the volume along the three orthogonal planes and use MagiCut to remove the obscuring areas (Figure 5.14)
Step 8:	The final rendered inverted version of the fetal heart may now be displayed as a 2D image in any color (Figure 5.15) or it seen as a cineloop of the beating heart

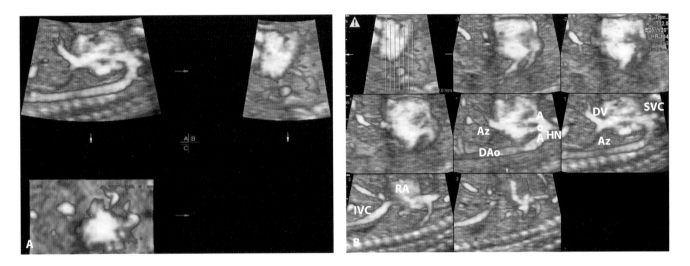

FIGURE 5.9 STIC volume of the heart of a 23w4d fetus with high-definition flow is acquired at an angle of 20 degrees starting from the sagittal plane. (A) Volume is displayed in the multiplanar mode. (B) Volume is displayed using TUI at a 2 mm interslice distance automatically generating all the required anatomical sagittal planes out of the single STIC volume. Note the aortic arch (AoA) descending aorta (DAo), head and neck vessels (HN), ductus venosus (DV), hypoechogenic azygous vein (Az) (no color uptake), right atrium (RA), and superior and inferior venae cavae (SVC and IVC).

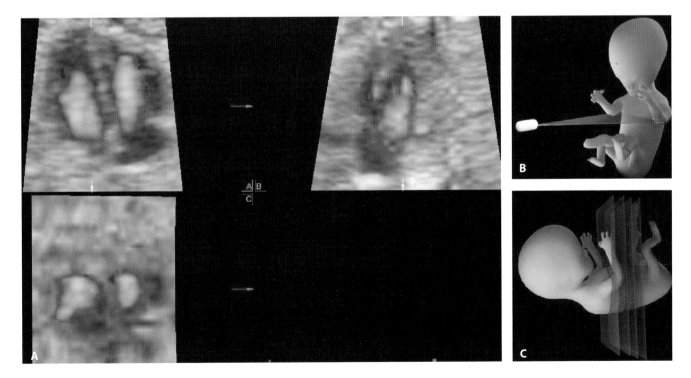

FIGURE 5.10 STIC acquisition. (A) STIC volume with high-definition flow of a 21w5d heart is acquired at an angle of 20 degrees. It is displayed in the multiplanar mode. (B) 3D model depicting the level of acquisition. (C) 3D model depicting the multiple overlaid 2D images. For a STIC, the volume would be limited to the heart.

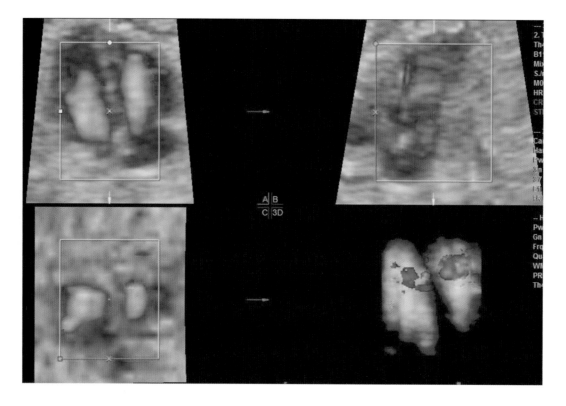

FIGURE 5.11 The same volume from Figure 5.11 is now rendered using surface rendering with the direction of the region of interest set at a back-to-front direction.

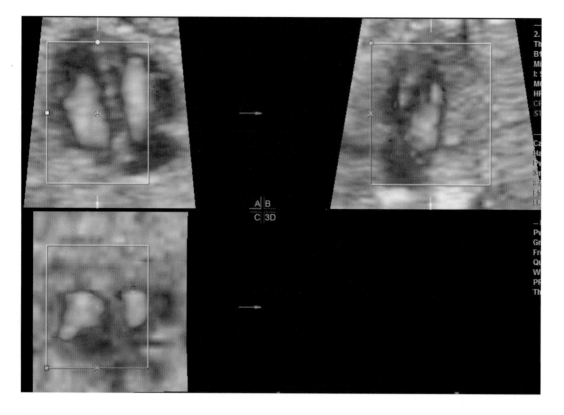

FIGURE 5.12 Render mode now changed to inversion. However, at the current settings no image is generated.

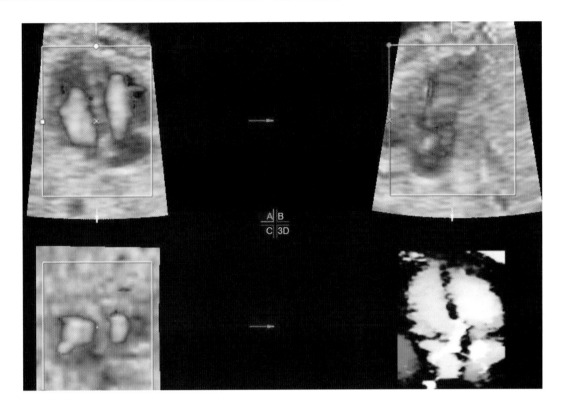

FIGURE 5.13 Mix and threshold settings are now adjusted, generating a cast of the fetal heart with the atrial and ventricular septae visible

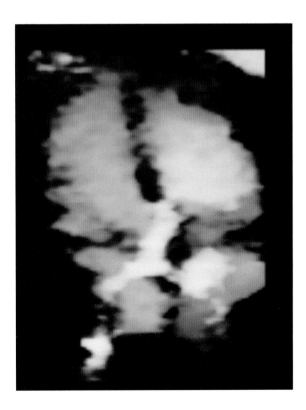

FIGURE 5.14 A single pane is now selected and the inverted heart, premanipulation, is shown.

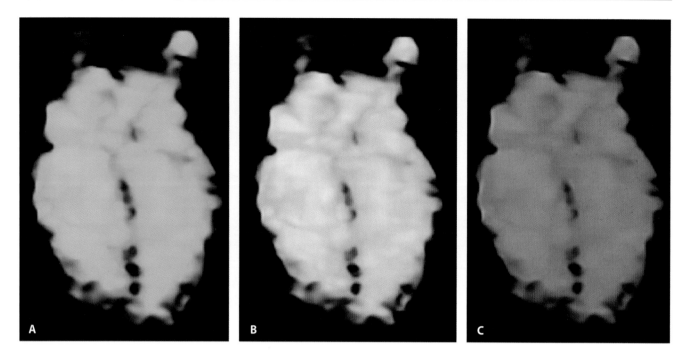

FIGURE 5.15 Postmanipulation. (A,B,C) Volume is now rotated along the three axes, and MagiCut is utilized to crop away any obscuring areas. Volume is displayed in various color settings. It may be viewed as a cineloop and rotated along any of the three axes. Care must be employed to not erroneously diagnose ventricular septal defects in this case, as these are rendering artifacts.

CONCLUSION

STIC is a unique 4D technique that enables full evaluation of the structure and function of the fetal heart, while it is beating, throughout a full cardiac cycle. It enables off-line study, review, and consultation on the most challenging fetal organ. Proper acquisition of the volume is key to facilitate navigation through it; however, it remains limited by the suboptimal resolution in the B and C planes.

PRACTICAL PEARLS

- STIC is a most useful modality for analyzing the fetal cardiac structure and function throughout a full cardiac cycle
- STIC enables visualization of ventricular filling during diastole and ventricular emptying during systole
- STIC allows a virtual cardiac examination and may be combined with other modalities such as TUI for a thorough multiplanar evaluation
- Remember to optimize the 2D settings prior to acquisition
- Avoid acquiring any volumes with fetal extremities covering the chest
- Use the smallest acquisition box and smallest angle possible to minimize artifacts

6 3D Tools

INTRODUCTION

Once a volume is acquired and displayed in either the multiplanar mode or in a rendered mode, several tools may be utilized to enhance the final images and facilitate the retrieval and evaluation of challenging areas. The availability of these modalities varies among manufacturers, and though many are standard, the given names are industry specific.

MagiCut

The electronic scalpel, MagiCut, is one of the most useful tools, allowing the sonologist to sculpt away and remove any structures that may be obscuring the area of interest. To use the MagiCut properly, the examiner must be aware of which structures within the volume are to be evaluated and which structures need to be removed. For optimal images, the volume can be rotated along the three axes to ascertain the depth and direction of the structures that need to be removed using the MagiCut tool. The main drawback is iatrogenic artifacts from excess removal by MagiCut, as this may generate artifacts that could distort the image, potentially alarming the patient. Figure 6.1 through Figure 6.4 depict before and after images where MagiCut was utilized (Table 6.1). On several of the newer machines, when the volume contains color Doppler there is an option to select whether to remove the gray-scale portion of the image, the color Doppler, or both when selecting a specific area within the volume.

VOLUME CONTRAST IMAGING

There are several slicing modalities that can be utilized for volume rendering in order to improve the visualization of the final rendered structure. One example is volume contrast imaging (VCI). This is a thick-slice technique where, instead of a thin 2D image display, a thick slice along an adjustable thickness may be obtained, minimizing artifacts and improving the quality of the image. VCI may be combined

Table 6.1 Steps to Using MagiCut

Step 1:	Obtain a 3D volume of a fetus and display it in the multiplanar mode selecting surface rendering (Figure 6.1)
Step 2:	Select the single image display to see the fetus in surface rendering (Figure 6.2)
Step 3:	Use the line or box, depending on the shape or the object to be removed, in order to remove what is obscuring the fetal details (Figure 6.3)
Step 4:	Adjust the threshold, render mode, and light to optimize the final rendered image (Figure 6.4)

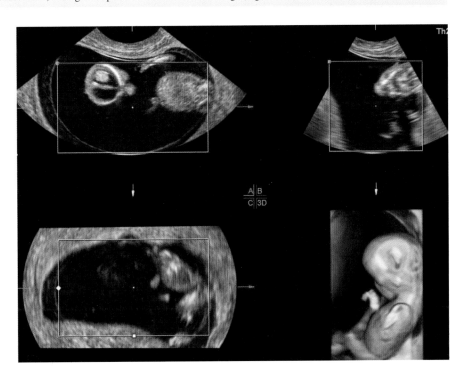

FIGURE 6.1 A 3D transvaginal volume of a 12-week fetus is obtained, displayed in the three orthogonal planes as well as surface rendering. Note the placenta anterior to the fetus in the rendered image.

with other modes, such as TUI. This aids in the visualization of certain structures within the brain, such as choroid plexus cysts, the cerebellar vermis, the corpus callosum (Figures 6.5–6.7), and the fetal spine. VCI is also helpful in evaluating the internal structures, such as the fetal heart and abdominal contents, as depicted in subsequent chapters.

OmniView

OmniView is a versatile slicing tool that allows slicing along any direction in a straight line or a curvilinear line. This may be accomplished utilizing various thicknesses, giving access to specific difficult-to-reach areas. It may be used as a single line or multiple lines within the same volume for various depictions. What is most unique about OmniView is that it allows the simultaneous display of three non-orthogonal planes from a single volume (Figure 6.8). There are several areas where OmniView is of great utility, such as in evaluating the fetal palate (Tonni et al. 2012) and the skeletal system as well as the internal organs. Further examples will be presented in the respective chapters.

VIRTUAL ORGAN COMPUTER-AIDED ANALYSIS

Virtual organ computer-aided analysis (VOCAL) is a 3D software that facilitates calculation of the volume of a specific area under study. This can be carried out by obtaining a volume of the area in question, such as a volume of the fetal lung. Tracing the structure of interest and rotating it along a 180-degree axis automatically calculates and generates the volume of the organ. This is of utmost utility in trying to determine the volume of the lungs, especially in the presence of congenital diaphragmatic hernia. It may also be used for the fetal liver, spleen, a particular mass, or even a fluid-filled area. Details on how to calculate the volume of a fetal lung are presented in Table 6.2 (Figures 6.9–6.12).

SonoAVC

SonoAVC is a specific volume calculation software that identifies several small echolucent areas and color codes them in order to distinguish them from one another. It is available

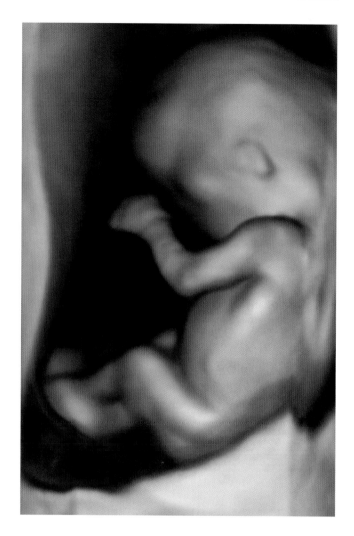

FIGURE 6.2 The rendered image is subsequently selected and the fetus rotated along the three orthogonal planes to depict as much of the entire fetus as possible. The volume now shows both feet.

as "SonoAVC follicle", which is to be used in reproductive medicine, or "SonoAVC general", which may be used everywhere else. The volume for the specific color-coded, identified areas may be calculated automatically. This has several applications: in the assessment of ovarian follicles (Table 6.3) (Figures 6.13–6.15), in the gastrointestinal and genitourinary tracts, and in the early developing fetal brain.

Table 6.2	**Steps to Using VOCAL for Calculating Lung Volume**
Step 1:	Obtain a 3D volume of the fetal chest and display it in the multiplanar mode (Figure 6.9).
Step 2:	Activate VOCAL. Select "manual" for the "define contour." Select "trace" for the "contour finder." Select a rotational step of 30 degrees. Select the reference image to carry out the measurements in (Figure 6.10)
Step 3:	With each rotation of the volume, trace around the visible portion of the corresponding lung (Figure 6.11)
Step 4:	In the case of a rotational step of 30 degrees, the system will prompt the sonographer to obtain 6 tracings. They would be a repetition of step 3 (Figure 6.11)
Step 5:	Once all 6 tracings have been carried out, select "done" and an automatic calculation of the volume with a 3D schematic will be displayed automatically (Figure 6.12)

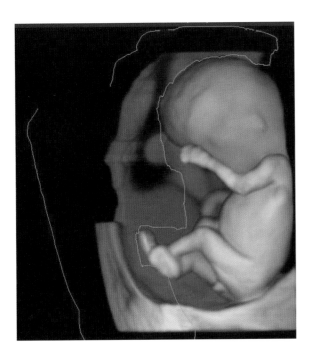

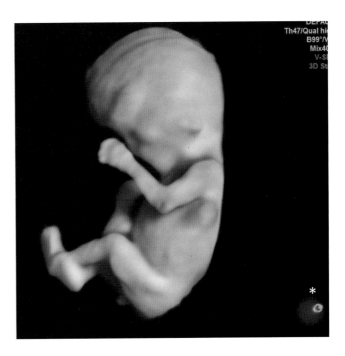

FIGURE 6.3 The volume is rotated along the *Y* axis and MagiCut is activated. MagiCut in this case employs "line trace" to remove areas "within" the line. The excess placental and other tissue is selected and removed.

FIGURE 6.4 This is the final volume after completing MagiCut. Further anticlockwise rotation is carried out along the *Y* axis. Finally, surface rendering is changed to HD*live*, and the threshold and light source are adjusted to generate this image. Note the orientation of the light source depicted in the schematic at the bottom right-hand corner of the image (*).

Table 6.3	**Steps to Using SonoAVC Follicle**
Step 1:	Obtain a 3D volume of the ovary
Step 2:	Select "SonoAVC follicle"
Step 3:	Automatically, all follicles (echolucent areas) get encircled and color coded (11 follicles in the volume in Figure 6.13 and Figure 6.14)
Step 4:	An automatic measurement in each of the 3 planes, together with the volume of each of the follicles, is then generated in a table (Figure 6.15)

FIGURE 6.5 A 3D volume of the fetal brain at 22w0d is displayed using TUI at an interslice thickness of 2 mm. Note where the interslice thickness is designated (*). The posterior fossa with the cerebellum (CB), thalami (Th), posterior horn of the lateral ventricle (Vp), falx cerebri (F), and cavum septi pellucidi (CSP) are seen.

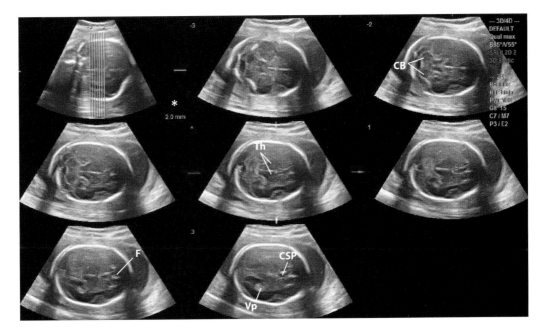

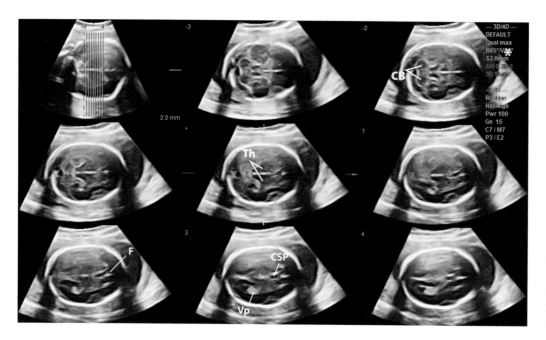

FIGURE 6.6 The same 3D volume of Figure 6.5 now displayed using VCI with a slice thickness of 2 mm (seen at the top right-hand corner [*]). The posterior fossa with the cerebellum (CB), thalami (Th), posterior horn of the lateral ventricle (Vp), falx cerebri (F), and cavum septi pellucidi (CSP) are seen. Note the improvement in the resolution and definition of the image.

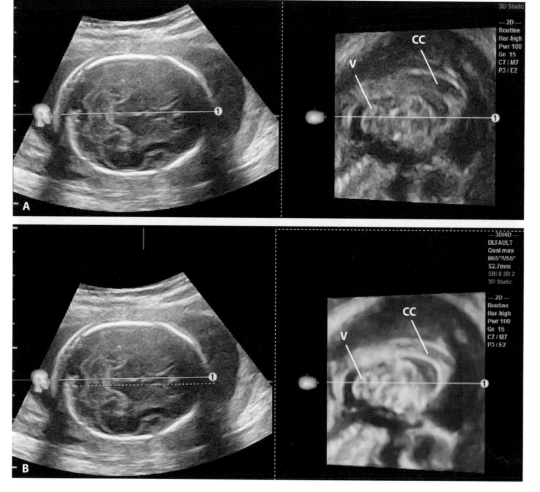

FIGURE 6.7 An axial 3D volume of the fetal brain at 22w0d. (A) OmniView is activated and a straight line is selected and it is drawn from posterior to anterior automatically generating a sagittal view of the corpus callosum (CC), a difficult plane to obtain. The cerebellar vermis is also seen (V). (B) VCI is now activated at a slice thickness of 2.7 mm and the color changed to sepia generating a clearer, crisper image.

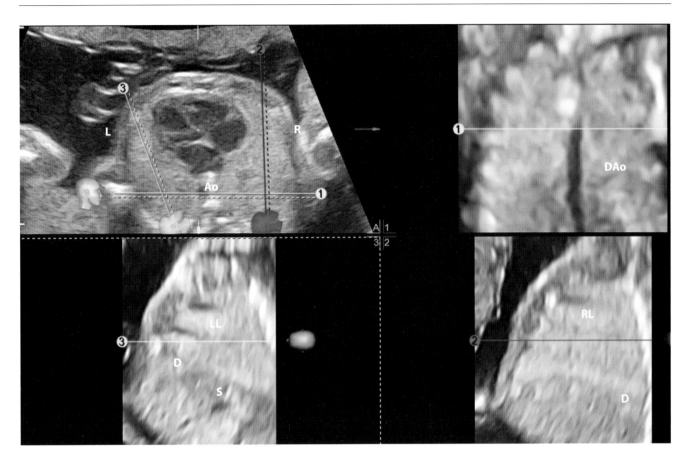

FIGURE 6.8 A 3D volume of a 21w5d fetal chest is obtained. The OmniView algorithm is employed with VCI at a slice thickness of 1 mm utilizing three color-coded polylines. The first line (1) is drawn from the left (L) to the right (R) of the chest across both lungs, transecting the aorta (Ao) in plane A. It generates an image of the descending aorta (DAo) in plane B. Line (2) is drawn from the posterior aspect of the right lung to the anterior abdominal wall, generating an image of the right lung (RL) with a clear diaphragm (D) seen in plane D. Line (3) is drawn from the posterior aspect of the left lung to the anterior abdominal wall, generating an image of the left lung (LL) with a clear diaphragm (D), and the stomach (S), seen in plane C.

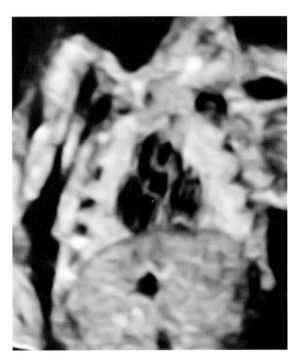

FIGURE 6.9 A 3D volume of the fetal chest and abdomen is obtained and displayed in the coronal plane utilizing VCI at a slice thickness of 2.5 mm.

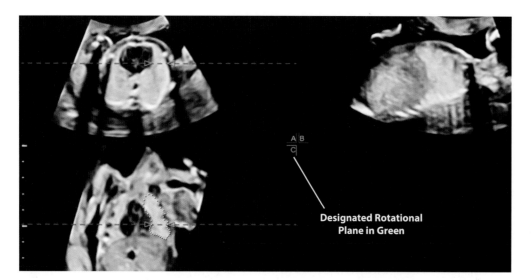

FIGURE 6.10 VOCAL is now activated and "manual" is selected for the "define contour" and "trace" for the "contour finder." A rotational step of 30 degrees is chosen. In this volume, plane C, the coronal plane, is the chosen reference plane in which to obtain the measurements. The dotted line in plane C depicts the first trace made of the area of the left lung.

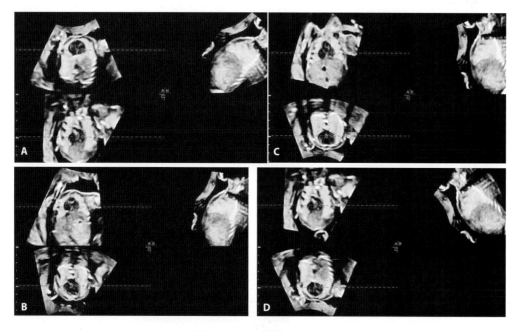

FIGURE 6.11 Rotational steps for VOCAL. (A–D) The system automatically generates a new plane for area-trace upon the completion of each of the six traces, as in this case of a 30-degree rotational step. Four of those planes are shown here.

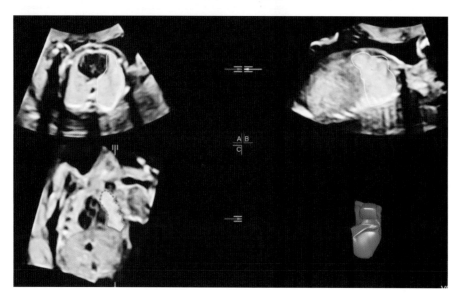

FIGURE 6.12 Once all six tracings have been carried out, "done" is selected. The area is highlighted in all three orthogonal planes, and an automatic calculation of the volume with a 3D schematic is displayed automatically.

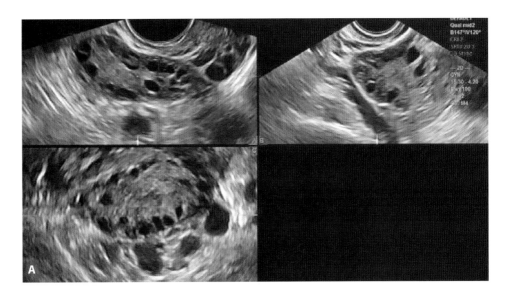

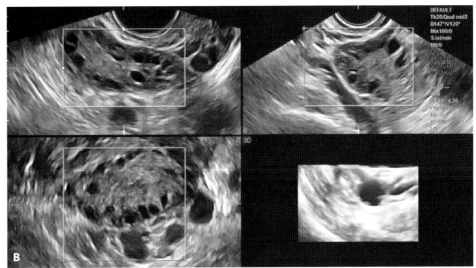

FIGURE 6.13 A SonoAVC follicle. (A) 3D transvaginal volume of the ovary is acquired, magnified, and displayed in the multiplanar mode. (B) SonoAVC follicle is selected, which automatically locates all the echolucent follicles and color-codes them.

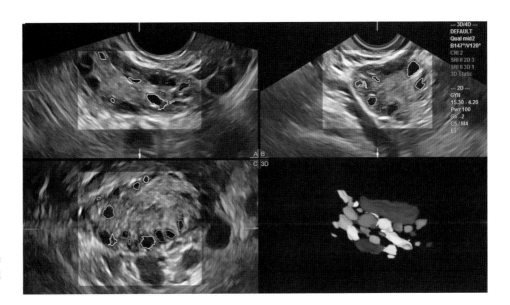

FIGURE 6.14 SonoAVC follicle has automatically identified and color-coded the follicles.

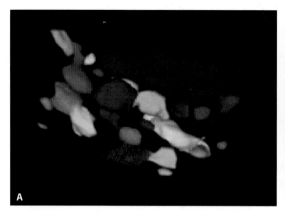

FIGURE 6.15 Volume calculation. (A) Various identified and color-coded follicles. (B) An automatic table is generated, depicting automatic measurements along the three axes, as well as automatic volume calculation, for each of the follicles, commencing with the largest. The data for the largest nine follicles are detailed in this example for the right ovary.

VOLUME COMPUTER-AIDED DIAGNOSIS

Volume computer-aided diagnosis (VCAD) is based on two main concepts, as described by Abuhamad (2004). The first concept states that any acquired volume contains within it all the 2D anatomical planes necessary for a complete assessment of the area in question. The second concept states that structures within that volume are organized in a constant relationship to each other.

Using VCAD, one can define the spatial relationships of any 2D planes of a particular organ in question, say the fetal heart, and then specific software may be utilized to automatically generate the specific 2D planes from the acquired volume in order to enable full assessment of the area in question. This has already been accomplished with the fetal heart, and the technique is described in a stepwise manner in Chapter 11. The same principles can be applied to any organ, such as the fetal brain or the first-trimester fetus (Abu-Rustum et al. 2012). The mid-sagittal volume technique for assessment of the first-trimester fetus is described in Chapter 7.

FRACTIONAL LIMB VOLUME

Fractional limb volume (FLV) is a novel sonographic tool based on the principle that fetal weight may be estimated from the limb volume (Lee et al. 2004, 2009). By obtaining a volume of the fetal thigh or arm, specific software may be employed which allows the sonographer to obtain several trace-measurements of the limb in question in order to calculate the fetal weight. This is described in detail in Chapter 15.

CONCLUSION

Once a volume is acquired, the sonographer may need to apply any combination of several tools to highlight the area under evaluation, remove obscuring structures, and employ modalities to help facilitate volume calculation and navigation within the volume. The applicability of these various tools is discussed further in the organ-specific chapters.

PRACTICAL PEARLS

- Several tools may be utilized to maximize the utility of volume sonography
- MagiCut allows sculpting and refining the image
- VCI allows for obtaining thick slices in the A and C planes
- In general, a VCI thickness of 2 mm is optimal for the study of the fetal brain (Chaoui oral communication 2013)
- It is recommended to utilize VCI on an already acquired volume rather than live, for optimal results (Chaoui oral communication 2013)
- It is possible to color-code the final image with respect to a particular application; for instance whenever TUI is utilized in a volume, the final image's color (whenever TUI is employed) may be set to copper or cool blue, or any other color (Chaoui oral communication 2013)
- OmniView allows any-direction linear and curvilinear multislicing within a volume at various thicknesses
- In general, an OmniView line set to a VCI slice thickness of 20 mm enables optimal evaluation of the fetal spine (Benoit oral communication 2012)
- VOCAL enables volume calculation of structures
- SonoAVC facilitates evaluation of multicystic/fluid-filled structures
- VCAD allows an assessment of the fetal heart and outflow tracts
- Fractional limb volume allows fetal weight estimation from a limb volume

7 Clinical Applicability in the First Trimester

INTRODUCTION

The applicability of volume sonography in the first trimester is unique in that a single volume of the entire fetus may be obtained in one sweep (Michailidis et al. 2002; Fauchon et al. 2008; Bharudi et al. 2010; Antsaklis et al. 2011; Borrell et al. 2011). From the volume it is possible to retrieve planes to evaluate fetal anatomy and measure the crown–rump length, limb lengths, biparietal diameter, head circumference, and abdominal circumference (Abu-Rustum et al. 2012).

CLINICAL UTILITY

There are several particular benefits to volume sonography in the first trimester and these are the focus of this chapter.

> ### BENEFITS OF VOLUME SONOGRAPHY IN THE FIRST TRIMESTER
>
> 1. Mid-sagittal volume technique for anatomic and biometric assessment
> 2. Single volume technique for evaluating the fetal heart
> 3. Volume NT
> 4. Sonoembryology

MID-SAGITTAL VOLUME TECHNIQUE

The mid-sagittal volume technique was described in 2012 (Abu-Rustum et al.) in which a single volume of the fetus is acquired along the mid-sagittal plane, the same plane utilized for measuring the nuchal translucency. First-trimester presets may be used and the volume may be acquired with an angle of acquisition of 65 degrees. Subsequent to that, the volume is standardized in plane A in order to depict the plane of the abdominal circumference in plane B, from which parallel shift is then utilized to navigate cephalad through the volume in order to visualize the fetal heart, upper limbs, facial bones, orbits, plane of the biparietal diameter, and the plane of the butterfly, and caudad in order to visualize the fetal kidneys, cord insertion, bladder, and lower limbs. Table 7.1 covers the steps of the mid-sagittal volume technique (Figures 7.1–7.14).

SINGLE-VOLUME TECHNIQUE TO EVALUATE THE FETAL HEART

With the small size of the fetal heart and the proximity of the 2D anatomical planes – the fetal stomach, four-chamber view, and three-vessel view – it is possible to examine these planes, as well as several other transverse cardiac planes, from a single volume. Using the first-trimester cardiac preset, it is possible to acquire a volume of at least 20 degrees at the level of the four-chamber view and employ color Doppler or HD-Flow (which may be superior to color Doppler for the smaller vessels in the first trimester). The volume may be displayed using TUI, which enables visualization of the plane of the abdominal circumference with a visible stomach (establishing fetal situs), as well as the planes of the four-chamber view and the three-vessel view in addition to several other transverse cardiac planes. Standardization of evaluating the first-trimester heart from a single volume using STIC modality with color Doppler was first described in 2009 (Turan et al.) and enables full cardiac assessment in up to 85% of fetuses (Table 7.2; Figures 7.15–7.18).

Table 7.1 **Steps for the Application of the Mid-Sagittal Volume Technique**

Step 1:	The volume is acquired from a sagittal plane with an angle of acquisition of 65 degrees (Figure 7.1)
Step 2:	The volume is then standardized in reference plane A via rotation along the X, Y, and Z axes to optimize the depiction of the fetus in the mid-sagittal plane (Figure 7.2)
Step 3:	In reference plane A, the reference dot is then placed on the fetal spine at the level of the diaphragm, automatically generating the axial plane of the fetal abdominal circumference, with a visible stomach, in plane B (Figure 7.3)
Step 4:	Plane B is then selected as the reference plane, and rotation along the Z axis is employed to optimize the location of the spine to 12 o'clock (Figure 7.4)
Step 5:	Parallel shift is then utilized to navigate cephalad within the volume, from reference plane B, to generate six anatomic planes (Figures 7.5–7.10)
Step 6:	Parallel shift is then utilized to navigate caudad within the volume, from reference plane B, to generate four anatomic planes (Figures 7.11–7.14)

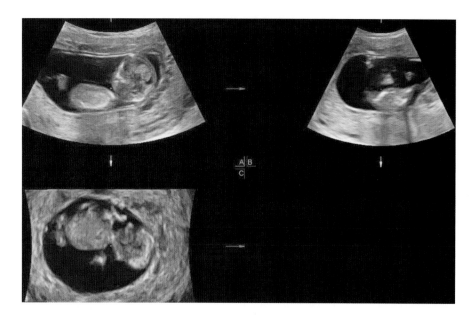

FIGURE 7.1 3D volume of a 13w1d fetus is acquired using first-trimester presets and an angle of acquisition of 65 degrees. The volume is displayed in the multiplanar mode, depicting all three orthogonal planes.

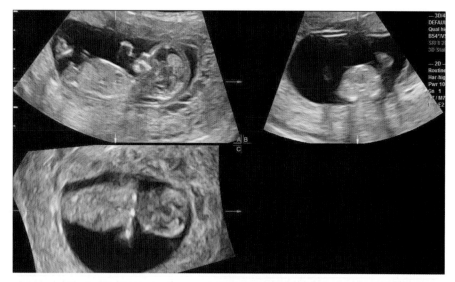

FIGURE 7.2 The volume is subsequently rotated along the *X, Y,* and *Z* axes in plane A to depict the fetus in as mid-sagittal a lie as possible, the same plane in which the nuchal translucency is measured.

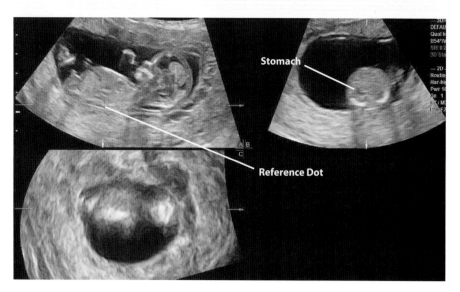

FIGURE 7.3 In plane A the reference dot moved to the fetal spine at the level of the diaphragm. This automatically generates the axial plane of the fetal abdominal circumference in plane B, with a visible stomach.

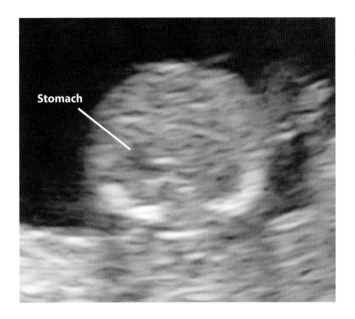

FIGURE 7.4 Plane B is then chosen as the reference plane from which to navigate cephalad and caudad within the volume using parallel shift.

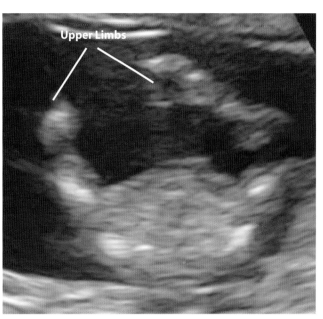

FIGURE 7.6 Scrolling further cephalad, it is possible to see the upper limbs.

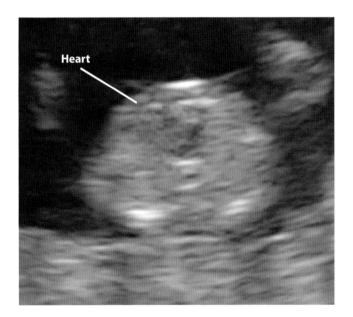

FIGURE 7.5 Scrolling cephalad from the plane of the abdominal circumference, the fetal heart is reached, and it is possible to ascertain situs.

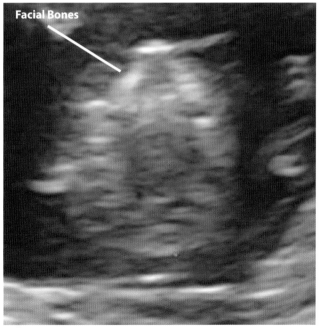

FIGURE 7.7 Scrolling further cephalad, it is possible to see the facial bones. Depending on the degree of flexion of the fetal head, it may also be possible to see the retronasal triangle, as is the case with this fetus.

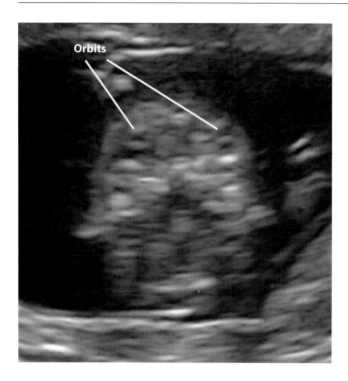

FIGURE 7.8 Scrolling further cephalad, the fetal orbits and even the lenses may be seen.

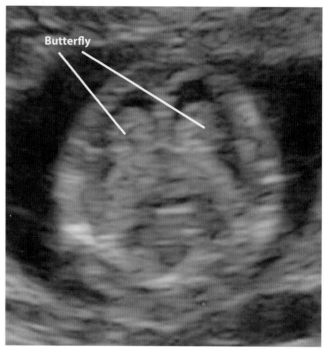

FIGURE 7.10 Further cephalad, the plane of the butterfly, formed by the choroid plexus filling the lateral ventricles, is reached.

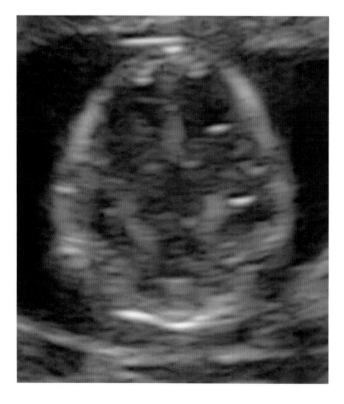

FIGURE 7.9 Scrolling further cephalad, the plane of the biparietal diameter is reached.

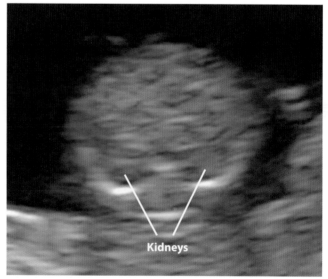

FIGURE 7.11 Scrolling caudad from the plane of the abdominal circumference, it is possible to visualize the fetal kidneys.

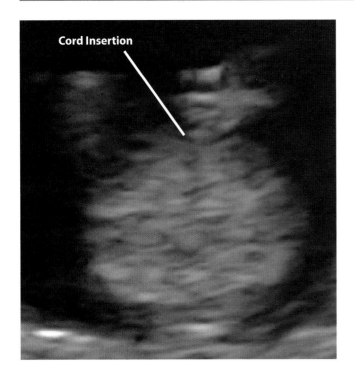

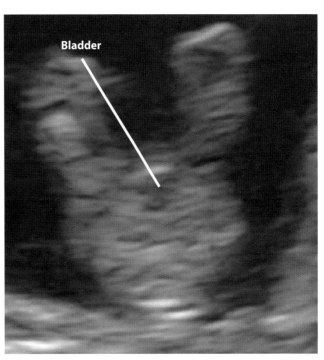

FIGURE 7.12 Scrolling further caudad, the cord insertion may be visualized.

FIGURE 7.13 Scrolling further caudad, the fetal bladder may be seen.

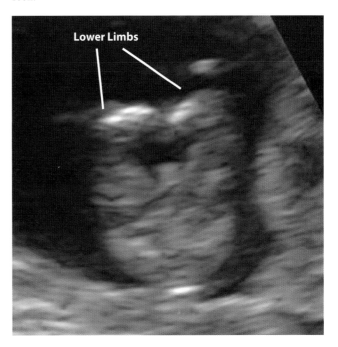

FIGURE 7.14 At the level of the bladder and scrolling even further caudad, the fetal lower limbs may be seen.

Table 7.2	**Steps for the Application of the Single Volume Technique for Evaluating the Fetal Heart**
Step 1:	The volume is acquired from a transverse plane at the level of the four-chamber view, with HD-Flow, using an angle of acquisition of 55 degrees (Figure 7.15)
Step 2:	The volume is then standardized in reference plane A via rotation along the Z axis in order to place the fetal spine at 6 o'clock and the cardiac apex to the left of the image (Figure 7.16)
Step 3:	In reference plane A, the reference dot is then placed at the crux of the heart (Figure 7.17)
Step 4:	Plane A is then selected as the reference plane and TUI at an interslice thickness of 1.2 mm and set to 15 slices is used to display the volume (Figure 7.18)
Step 5:	From the displayed volume, the planes of the abdominal circumference with a visible stomach, the four-chamber and three-vessel view become apparent (Figure 7.18)

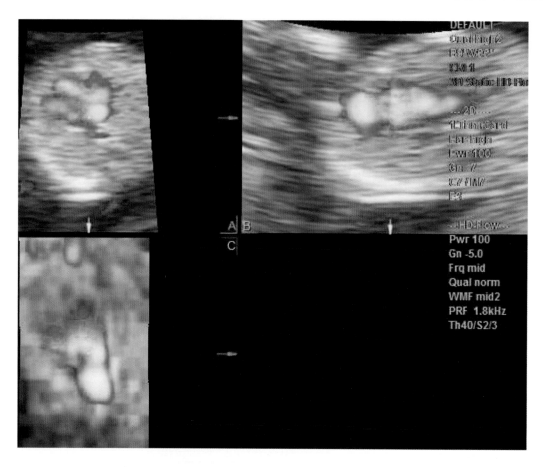

FIGURE 7.15 3D volume is acquired at the level of the four-chamber view, after the application of HD-Flow, using first trimester cardiac presets and an angle of acquisition of 55 degrees. The volume is subsequently displayed in the multiplanar view depicting all three orthogonal planes.

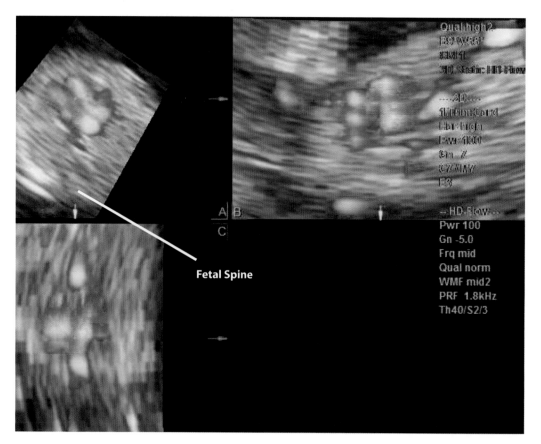

FIGURE 7.16 The volume is then standardized in plane A by rotation along the Z axis in order to place the fetal spine in the 6 o'clock position.

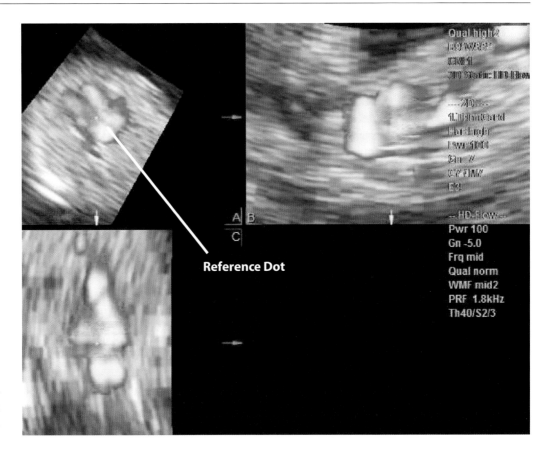

FIGURE 7.17 The reference dot is then placed at the crux of the heart in plane A.

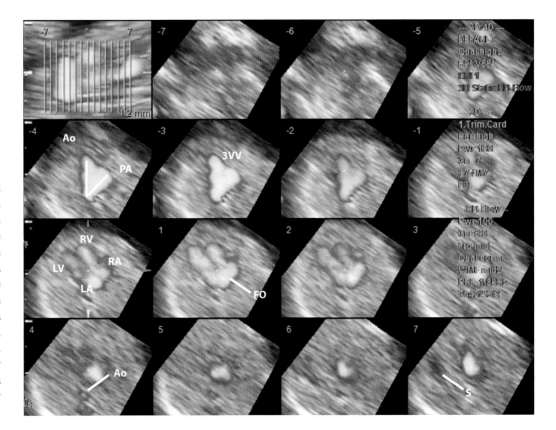

FIGURE 7.18 The volume is then displayed using TUI set at 15 slices 1.2 mm apart. Through this display, it is possible to see the fetal stomach (S), the left-sided aorta in cross-section (Ao), the four-chamber view with the ventricles and atria (RV, LV, RA, and LA), the foramen ovale (FO), and the three-vessel view (3VV) with the aorta (Ao) and pulmonary artery (PA).

Volume Nuchal Translucency

Volume nuchal translucency (NT) is a specific volume-based software available on select ultrasound machines in which a volume of the first-trimester fetus is acquired in the mid-sagittal plane. After acquisition of the volume and using the applicable presets on the machine, there is automatic generation of an optimized, magnified mid-sagittal image of the fetal head and thorax (Figure 7.19). Subsequently, the operator places a box over the optimal area for measuring the NT for automatic generation of the fetal NT.

Sonoembryology

Another in vivo application for volume sonography in the first trimester is to facilitate the study of the fetal ventricular system (Figure 7.20). This requires expertise and a clear understanding of fetal embryology. By applying the inversion mode, and possibly employing SonoAVC to volumes of the developing fetal brain, a cast of the fetal ventricular system may be obtained and it can be studied at various gestations, as has been described by Kim et al. (2008), for the potential early recognition and identification of underlying central nervous system abnormalities.

Limitations of Volume Sonography in the Evaluation of the First-Trimester Fetus

Although volume sonography has great advantages in the first trimester, facilitated by the ability to obtain a single volume of the entire fetus for later off-line analysis, there remain several limitations. At this point in gestation the fetus is often in a flexed position, with the upper limbs obscuring the face. In addition, there tends to be significant fetal motion beyond 13 weeks, resulting in artifact introduction. As a result, the optimal time for volume acquisition is after 12 weeks, when the fetus is in a near-still sagittal lie. One must also keep in mind the developmental limitations, such as normal fetal gut herniation, in order to avoid misdiagnoses which could cause undue parental anxiety.

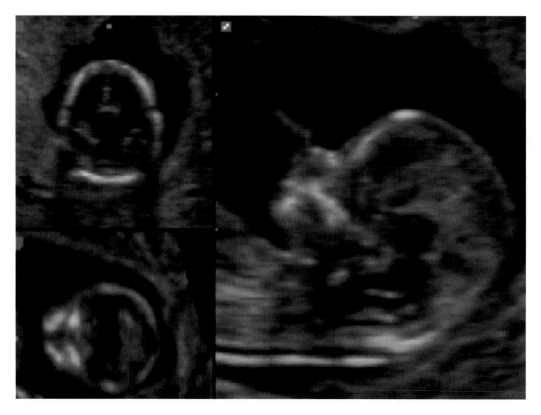

FIGURE 7.19 Using volume NT, available on select ultrasound machines, a 3D volume of the fetal head and upper chest is acquired in the mid-sagittal plane. After the acquisition of the volume and using the applicable presets on the machine, there is the automatic generation of an optimized, magnified mid-sagittal image of the fetal head and thorax (right-hand image) with the corresponding orthogonal planes depicted in the two left-hand images.

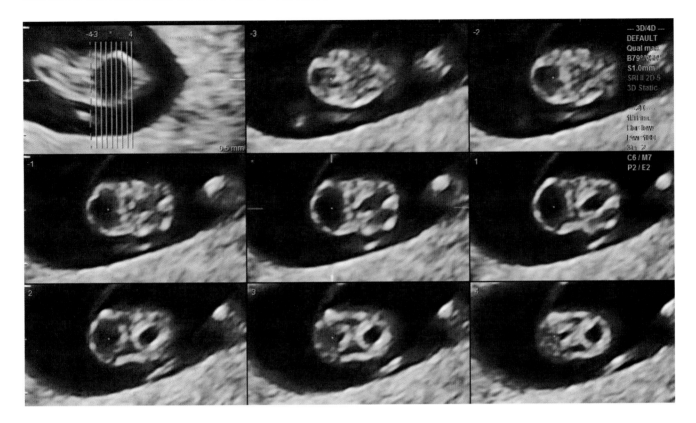

FIGURE 7.20 A transvaginal volume of an 8w4d fetus is acquired and displayed using TUI at an interslice thickness of 0.5 mm and with VCI at a slice thickness of 1 mm depicting the developing ventricular system.

CONCLUSION

The proper application of volume sonography in the first trimester facilitates the complete fetal anatomic and biometric assessment from a single volume acquired in a mid-sagittal plane (Figure 7.21) (Abu-Rustum et al. 2012). With the proper acquisition and display of a single volume of the first-trimester fetal heart utilizing HD-Flow, it may also be possible to generate most of the transverse cardiac planes necessary for the evaluation of the fetal heart. Off-line analysis of first-trimester of fetal brain volumes utilizing the various 3D modalities such as the inversion mode may enhance the comprehension of fetal development. As technology evolves, automation may ultimately enable a full first-trimester fetal assessment by generating all of the anatomic and biometric first-trimester planes required for evaluation of the first-trimester fetus. With the introduction of noninvasive prenatal testing, it is inevitable that the role of the first-trimester scan will shift from screening for aneuploidy to a full fetal anatomic evaluation (Abu-Rustum 2014).

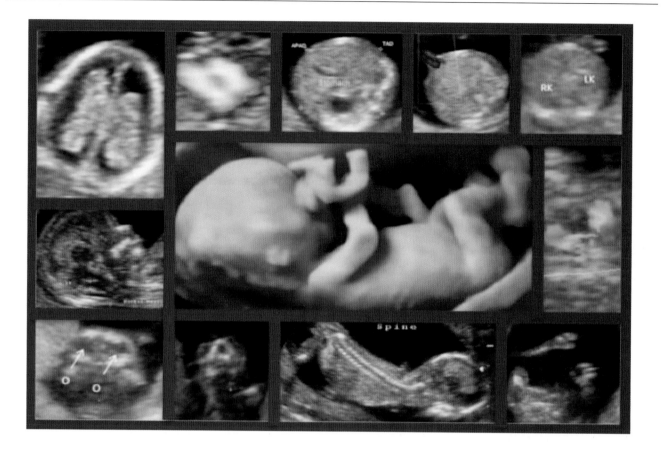

FIGURE 7.21 From a single 3D volume of a first-trimester fetus, it is possible to generate all the planes required for an anatomic and biometric assessment (RK and LK, right and left kidneys; O, orbits).

PRACTICAL PEARLS

- To maximize the success of retrieving all the respective anatomic and biometric planes out of a single volume, start with as true a mid-sagittal lie as possible, optimize the 2D settings, acquire the volume with an angle of 65 degrees
- Standardize the volume at the level of the abdominal circumference plane and scroll cephalad as well as caudad for a full assessment of the fetus in the first trimester
- For evaluating the fetal heart, acquire a 3D volume starting at the level of the four-chamber view using HD-Flow with an angle of acquisition of 55 degrees
- Display the volume using TUI at 12-15 slices 1.2–2 mm apart in order to establish fetal situs by visualizing the plane of the abdominal circumference as well as the planes of the four-chamber view and the three-vessel view

- It is possible to automatically generate the plane for measuring the fetal NT out of an acquired volume and to utilize specific software to automatically measure the optimal NT using certain sonographic machines
- Applying the inversion mode to a volume of the first trimester fetal brain allows the generation of a cast of the fetal ventricular system
- In the first trimester and with the small size of the fluid-filled structures, it may be easier to utilize SonoAVC follicle (Benoit oral communication 2012) to invert key structures in the brain and abdomen
- VCI is most helpful in the analysis of a first trimester volume

8 Clinical Applicability in the Fetal Face

INTRODUCTION

Nowhere is the beauty of volume sonography more apparent than in the evaluation of the fetal face, especially today with the availability of HD*live* (Figure 8.1). The fetal face is an area where 3D ultrasound has been proven to be of added clinical value in comparison to 2D sonography. In 1995 Devonald et al. described quasi-3D imaging as complementary to 2D imaging in the evaluation of the fetal face (Devonald et al. 1995), followed by Merz et al.'s report using transabdominal and transvaginal 3D ultrasound to detect or exclude facial abnormalities in 618 fetuses between 9 and 37 weeks. Merz concluded that 3D ultrasound provided convincing evidence for its use in the evaluation of normal and abnormal fetal anatomy (Merz et al. 1997). However, imaging of the fetal face has been one of the main reasons for the improper utilization of volume sonography for "entertainment ultrasound," and has resulted in abuse by some sonographers and physicians who have capitalized on the emotional component of 3D imaging. The purpose of this chapter is to demonstrate the value of 3D ultrasound beyond just the "pretty face," where much skill needs to be acquired and many techniques need to be mastered to use volume sonography to its fullest potential in evaluating the fetal face.

CLINICAL UTILITY

Volume sonography has been shown to be of added utility in identifying several abnormalities of the fetal face, the most common areas of which are listed below. Please refer to Chapter 2, where Table 2.2 and Figure 2.3 and 2.4 cover the basic steps for acquiring a volume of the fetal face.

FACIAL ABNORMALITIES WHERE VOLUME SONOGRAPHY IS OF ADDED VALUE

1. Facial clefts
2. Facial tumors
3. Orbital abnormalities
4. Nasal abnormalities
5. Maxillary/mandibular abnormalities
6. Neck abnormalities
7. Other

FACIAL CLEFTS

While the patient and family members are eager to see the fetal face, imaging of this structure by the physician is important to exclude facial abnormalities that at times may be isolated or may present as part of a syndrome. The area that has been studied extensively, using 3D ultrasound, is the prenatal diagnosis of facial clefting. Although a cleft lip can be easily visualized by surface rendering after artifactual shadowing has been excluded from the cord, placenta, limbs, or digits (Figure 8.2), the hard and soft palate prove to be much more difficult to image.

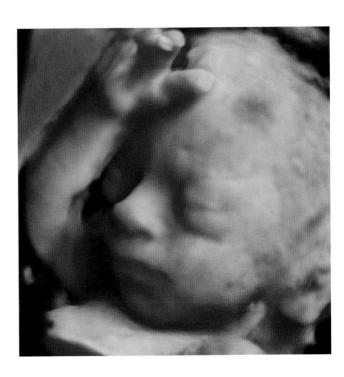

FIGURE 8.1 3D volume of a 23w6d fetus rendered using HD*live*. Note the details of the face: the eyelids, philtrum, and nostrils.

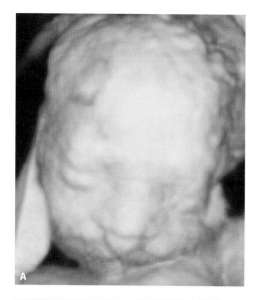
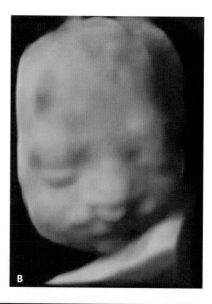

FIGURE 8.2 3D volume of a 26w6d fetus with bilateral cleft lip. (A) Volume is rendered using surface mode. (B) Volume is rendered using HD*live*. These images helped clarify the findings to the family.

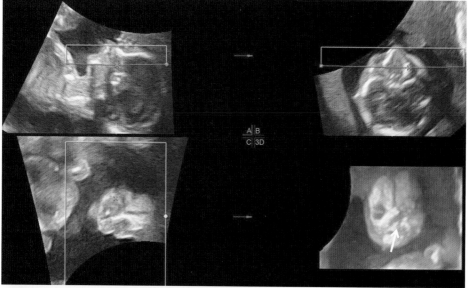

FIGURE 8.3 3D volume of a 19w0d fetus with a cleft palate is displayed in the multiplanar mode using skeletal mode. The reverse-face technique is utilized, clarifying the presence of the cleft palate (arrow).

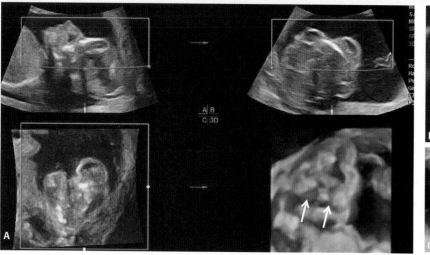
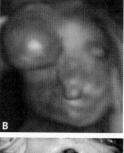
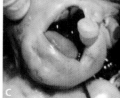

FIGURE 8.4 3D volume of a 20w4d fetus with multiple anomalies. (A) Volume is displayed in the multiplanar mode using skeletal mode. The reverse-face technique is used to show bilateral deep cleft palates (arrows). (B) Volume is displayed using surface mode, clearly depicting a frontal encephalocele, which mimics an orbital tumor and left exophthalmos. These images helped clarify the complex anomalies to the family. (C) Postmortem image confirming the findings of a deep right cleft lip and palate, a left cleft lip and palate, and left exophthalmos. The encephalocele ruptured during delivery (postnatal image courtesy of Adba Frangieh, MD).

FIGURE 8.5 The same 19w0d fetus as in Figure 8.3, evaluated using the flipped-face technique, where the image in plane A has now been flipped upside-down by 90 degrees. The cleft in the alveolar ridge and hard palate is visualized (arrow).

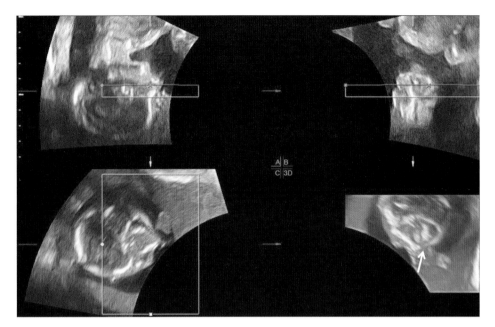

FIGURE 8.6 3D volume of a 22w6d fetus with an intact palate is evaluated using the OmniView algorithm with VCI. Here three polylines are used which facilitate the simultaneous display of three nonorthogonal planes, showing the uvula (U) and intact hard palate (HP).

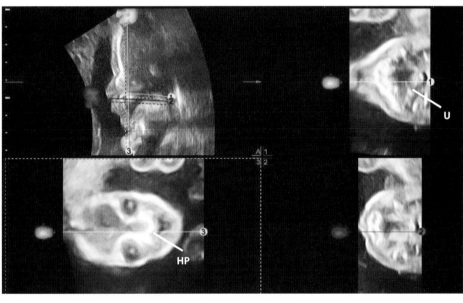

The clinician can use several imaging approaches to identify the facial structures such as the reverse-face (Figure 8.3 and 8.4), flipped-face (Figure 8.5), OmniView (Figure 8.6), oblique face, or a modification of all the above. The gold standard for the proper technique has yet to be established. Additional key points to keep in mind are how to acquire the image plane for evaluation of the fetal face. Options include the standard mid-sagittal view, the axial or coronal view.

The reverse-face technique was described by Campbell and Lees (2003) (Table 8.1). In this technique, an attempt is made to acquire a volume commencing from the sagittal plane, display it in the multiplanar mode, and then rotate the image in plane A by 180 degrees along the vertical Y axis. The render box is subsequently placed in the back-to-front orientation to visualize the palate by scrolling through the volume. The benefit of this technique is avoiding any shadowing anteriorly from a limb, the cord, or the placenta. In 2005, Campbell et al. reported on the use of this technique in eight cases of facial clefting (Campbell et al. 2005) with a high degree of diagnostic accuracy. However, a cleft in the soft palate was missed in one case.

In 2004, Rotten carried out a systemic analysis of the fetal face on 10,500 fetuses. Using 2D, a true mid-sagittal plane was acquired, and subsequently a coronal view, for a thorough evaluation of the fetal face. However, using 3D and 4D allowed for an easier, more rapid, and more accurate assessment of the normal fetal face (Rotten and Levaillant 2004a). Rotten then carried out one of the largest case series, on 96 fetuses with various facial clefts. This was a retrospective review in which it was demonstrated that 3D/4D was superior to non-3D/4D imaging (Rotten and Levaillant 2004b).

Table 8.1 **Steps to Applying the Reverse-Face Technique**

Step 1:	Obtain a mid-sagittal view of the fetal face after optimizing all the 2D parameters using the surface-rendering mode (Figure 8.7 and 8.8)
Step 2:	Change the direction of viewing the region of interest to "back-to-front" (Figure 8.9)
Step 3:	The hard palate should now be visible in plane C (Figure 8.9)
Step 4:	The render mode, threshold, and various settings may be adjusted to optimize the final rendered image (Figure 8.10 and 8.11)

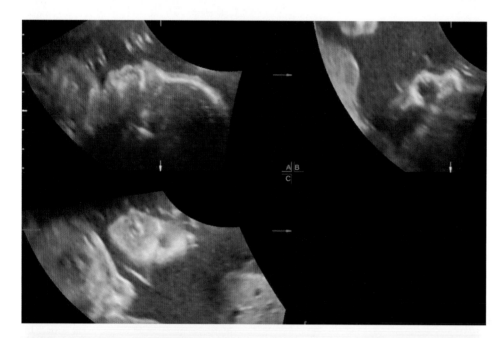

FIGURE 8.7 3D volume of a 22w2d fetus with a cleft lip is obtained, rotated along the three orthogonal planes to depict the fetus in a sagittal plane in plane A.

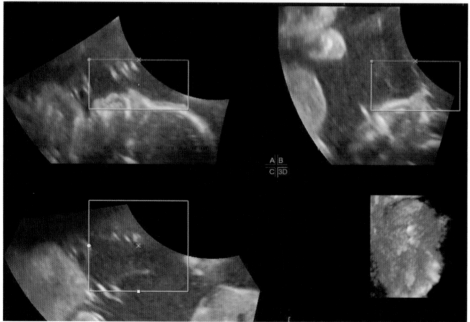

FIGURE 8.8 The same 3D volume of the 22w2d fetus in Figure 8.7 is now rendered using x-ray mode.

In the flipped-face technique described by Platt in 2006 (Table 8.2), a 3D volume is obtained with the fetus in the supine position and displayed in the multiplanar mode. Subsequently, the image in plane A is flipped by 90 degrees so that the fetus is now vertical with the chin up. The render box is then placed over the mandible, the size minimized to enhance resolution, and the volume is scrolled through from the chin to the nose. The main limitation in this technique is acquisition without

shadowing. As with the reverse-face technique, the ability to visualize the soft palate is limited (Platt et al. 2006).

Benacerraf et al., in 2006, described a case of Fryn's syndrome in which the fetus had multiple abnormalities. Here, 3D and fetal magnetic resonance imaging (MRI) were employed. Using the en-face thick-slice (VCI) technique, a cleft palate was detected which proved key to the prenatal diagnosis of Fryn's syndrome (Benacerraf et al. 2006).

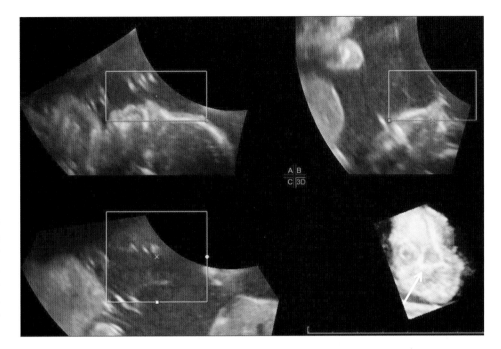

FIGURE 8.9 The direction of the render box for the fetus in Figure 8.8 is changed so that it is now back-to-front, with the settings optimized for visualizing the bony structures. This allows ascertaining the intactness of the alveolar ridge (arrow).

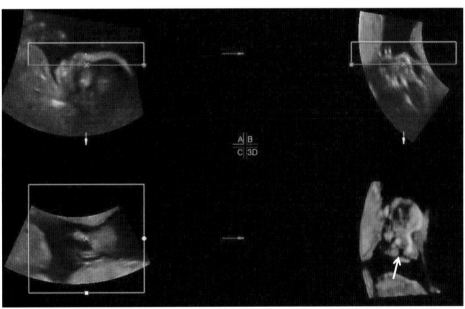

FIGURE 8.10 This is another example of the reversed-face technique on a 21w5d fetus with a cleft palate clearly visualized in the final rendered image in plane D (arrow).

In 2007 Faure introduced yet another technique, anterior axial 3D view, seen from the underside to visualize the secondary palate. The key differentiating factor for this technique is that the volume is acquired from the axial and not the mid-sagittal plane, as in the previously described reversed- or flipped-face techniques. In the prospective study, Faure assessed 100 fetuses at 17, 22, 27, and 32 weeks. With the transducer just in front of the alveolar ridge, all aspects of the posterior palate were studied by visualizing seven defined anatomic landmarks. Sonographic findings were subsequently compared to surgical fetopathological specimens. The ideal time for utilizing this technique was determined to be at 20–24 weeks (Faure et al. 2007).

Pilu described a novel technique for the palate: angle of insonation with 3D. This technique was used in 15 normal fetuses at 19–28 weeks and one fetus with a cleft at 33 weeks (Pilu and Segata 2007). The main goal of this technique was to insonate at a 45-degree angle to avoid shadowing from the alveolar ridge. The modes used were the multiplanar, surface display (maximum mode) in addition to TUI and VCI. The authors concluded that in normal fetuses, the axial and coronal acquisitions were as helpful, but in the abnormal cases, the coronal acquisition proved to be more helpful. However, the authors remained uncertain as to this technique's utility in isolated clefts of the soft palate.

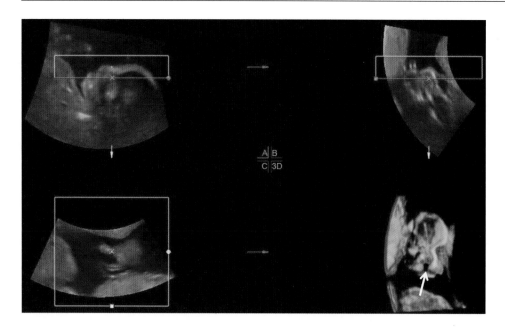

FIGURE 8.11 The same 21w5d fetus from Figure 8.10 in which the image mix settings have been adjusted further, enabling ascertainment of the cleft palate.

Table 8.2 **Steps to Applying the Flipped-Face Technique**

Step 1:	Obtain a volume starting from the mid-sagittal view of the face utilizing the surface-rendering mode as was done for the "reverse-face" technique (Figure 8.12)
Step 2:	Place the reference dot just below the philtrum (Figure 8.12)
Step 3:	Rotate the image in plane A around the Z axis by 90 degrees (Figure 8.13)
Step 4:	Place the render box over the mouth and adjust its size to encompass the bony area under examination (Figure 8.13)
Step 5:	Scroll through the axial plane and adjust the render mode in order to see the lips, alveolar ridge, mandible, maxilla, and hard and soft palates (Figure 8.14)

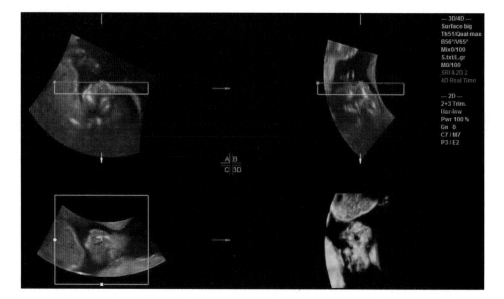

FIGURE 8.12 The same 21w5d fetus previously examined using the reverse-face technique, now examined using the flipped-face technique. The initial steps are the same, with an acquired volume displayed in the maximum mode starting with a sagittal plane in plane A. The reference dot is placed just below the philtrum.

McGahan et al. in 2008 used the 3D multislice display (TUI) to help identify facial clefts. The technique was standardized in both the axial and sagittal planes. This enabled full visualization of the fetal face from the palate to the orbits in nine slices, where the interslice thickness was set at 3.7 mm (McGahan et al. 2008).

In 2008 Zoppi et al. reported on an isolated case of a cleft palate in a high-risk patient who had been missed on routine sonographic evaluation. However, re-evaluation of the stored volume, using an axial 3D reconstruction, enabled visualization of the cleft (Zoppi et al. 2008). From this report, one can infer that even if an isolated cleft palate is missed on routine evaluation, if there is a suspicion of a cleft palate, the

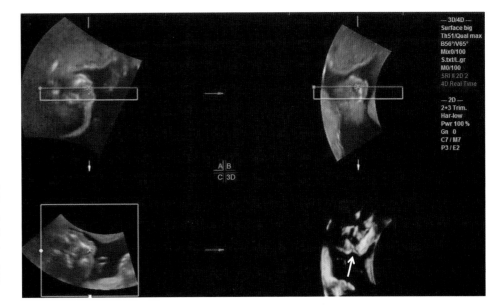

FIGURE 8.13 Post acquisition, the image in plane A is rotated along the Z axis by 90 degrees. The reference box is minimized in size to generate a view of the palate which clearly depicts the cleft, starting with the alveolar ridge and extending inward (arrow).

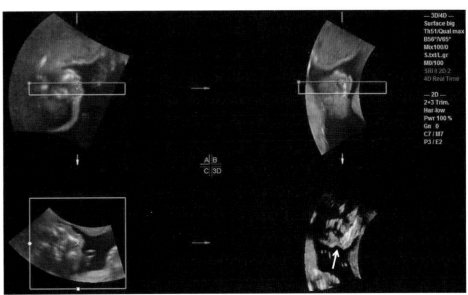

FIGURE 8.14 The image mix settings are changed from Figure 8.13 to examine the cleft palate further.

examiner could carry an off-line re-examination of the volume, utilizing all the available techniques, to further determine the presence or absence of a cleft palate. If that were to be confirmed, the parents would be re-contacted to make the necessary arrangements for follow-up and further care and management.

Faure et al. in 2008 noted that the arching of the soft palate puts it in a different plane than the hard palate, which contributes to the inadequacy of its visualization. They suggested that this can be avoided by employing the 30 degree, 3D-inclined axial view. This was evaluated on 87 low-risk fetuses at 21–25 weeks, in which a volume was obtained for examination of the soft palate. The images were subsequently compared to pathological specimens. Although this technique's reproducibility was not evaluated, it was found to be of utility in assessing intactness of the soft palate (Faure et al. 2008).

As a result of the availability of so many different techniques with which to evaluate the face, a study was carried out by Martínez Ten in 2009 to compare the various techniques for visualization of the soft palate (Martínez Ten et al. 2009). Ten fetuses with clefts and 50 normal fetuses, at 20–33 weeks of gestation, were evaluated. The authors concluded that in order to visualize the soft palate, a near-perfect volume must be obtained with a good fluid interphase between the fetal tongue and palate. The oblique and flipped-face techniques proved to be the superior techniques.

In 2009 Wong et al. re-examined the fetal palate from stored volumes of 31 normal fetuses at 15–35 weeks. It was determined that visualizing the uvula, which corresponds to the soft palate, is most difficult at less than 19 weeks and beyond 35 weeks, when the angulation of the arch is even greater, putting it in a more difficult plane to access in comparison to the plane of the hard palate (Wong et al. 2009).

Most recently, in 2012 Tonni et al. reported on the "OmniView Algorithm" as a new 3D technique for the study of the fetal hard and soft palates, in which it is possible to simultaneously display three nonorthogonal planes commencing from a fetus in a mildly flexed position (Tonni et al. 2012). Ideally, there needs to be fluid in the oropharynx and the absence of the cord or limbs from in front of the face. Here, skeleton mode is used to acquire the volume from the top of the head to the chin, using an angle of roughly 65 degrees. The OmniView algorithm is then employed utilizing three polylines. The first line is drawn from the posterior aspect of the palate down to the chin, generating an image of the labia, alveolar ridge, and the uvula (indicating an intact palate). The second line is drawn from the anterior and posterior nasal spines to the tip of the uvula. This generates an image that shows the labia and alveolar ridge. The third is a vertical line extending behind the frontal bone down to the chin, the equivalent of the reverse mode. This generates an image of the hard palate and tongue (Figure 8.6).

In summary, the ideal technique for the evaluation of the fetal face for the various types of clefts has yet to be ascertained. For this reason, it is important to be aware of all the available techniques and when indicated, whether because of history, current suspicion, or the mere presence of a cleft lip, to employ these various modalities in an attempt to ascertain intactness or involvement of the hard and soft palates.

FACIAL TUMORS

There is a multitude of facial tumors where volume sonography has been utilized to further characterize the mass in question, and to aid in planning the intrapartum and postpartum care of these babies. One of the earliest reports was by Shaw et al. in 2004 in a case of congenital epulis, a gingival granular cell tumor. In this case, 3D aided in the visualization of the mass; however, it was misleading in giving the impression that an EXIT procedure was needed, where in reality it was not (Shaw et al. 2004). An EXIT procedure (ex utero intrapartum treatment) is performed at the time of cesarean delivery whenever fetal airway obstruction is suspected. Using EXIT, the fetal airway is secured prior to clamping the umbilical cord.

CLINICAL UTILITY OF VOLUME SONOGRAPHY IN FACIAL TUMORS

1. Sizing of the tumor
2. Assessing extent of airway involvement and determining the need for an EXIT procedure

In 2005 Paladini et al. used volume sonography on a cavernous hemangioma of the face and neck. This was of utmost utility in counseling the family, and in consultation with the surgeons to plan care for this fetus (Paladini et al. 2005).

Another report on a palatal teratoma by Merhi et al. in 2005 concluded that 3D and color Doppler helped clarify the extent of the teratoma, which may have been missed by 2D, and determined that there was no need for an EXIT procedure. This facilitated planning of intrapartum/postpartum care (Merhi et al. 2005). In contrast, Shih et al. reported on the use of 3D and MRI in the case of an oral tumor, an epignathus, and in this case it helped prepare for an EXIT procedure by clarifying the extent of the tumor and the obstruction to the airway (Shih et al. 2005). Sherer et al. reported a similar case in 2006 where, again, 3D of a massive fetal epignathus helped in the decision regarding an EXIT procedure by delineating the extent of the tumor (Sherer et al. 2006).

ORBITAL ABNORMALITIES

Although orbital abnormalities (Figure 8.4) are not that common, they do carry serious implications. In 2000, Blaas et al. reported on a nine-week fetus with holoprosencephaly, cyclopia, and a proboscis (Figure 8.15) using transvaginal scan "any plane" 3D slicing technique. This enabled reconstruction of facial planes otherwise unavailable through 2D and provided valuable additional information (Blaas et al. 2000b).

CLINICAL UTILITY OF VOLUME SONOGRAPHY IN ORBITAL ABNORMALITIES

1. Ascertaining the presence of cyclopia, anophthalmia
2. Ascertaining the presence and extent of dacrocystoceles

Sepulveda et al. reported on 10 cases of congenital dacrocystocele. In 3/10 cases, volume sonography was used and helped clarify the abnormality. This was in terms of the extent of the dacrocystocele's extension into the nasal cavity as well as any connection between the nasal cavity and the orbits. The results were comparable to MRI and deemed worthy of considering 3D as the standard for scanning in these cases (Sepulveda et al. 2005).

Johnson et al. used 3D in a case of oculoauricularfrontonasal syndrome. In this case, 3D provided invaluable information to the couple in appreciating the abnormality (Johnson et al. 2005).

Most recently, Wong et al. used the reverse-face view to visualize a case of anophthalmia. The benefit of this technique was in eliminating the shadows and clarifying the abnormality (Wong et al. 2008).

NASAL ABNORMALITIES

The presence or absence of the nasal bone, as well as its hypoplasia, in the first and second trimesters has great implications in the fetus' risk assessment for trisomies. Rembouskos et al. evaluated the role of volume sonography in determining the presence or absence of the fetal nasal bone. It was found that the key to ascertaining its presence was the initial 2D image, as utilizing 3D alone in cases of a suboptimal angle of acquisition may lead to false-positives (Rembouskos et al. 2004).

> ### CLINICAL UTILITY OF VOLUME SONOGRAPHY IN EVALUATING THE FETAL NOSE
>
> 1. Ascertaining the presence of both nasal bones utilizing the maximum mode
> 2. Measuring the width of the nasal bone gap in first trimester fetuses

To overcome the limitation of ascertaining the presence of the fetal nasal bone utilizing volume sonography, Benoit and Chaoui employed 3D maximum mode in assessing the presence of the fetal nasal bone (Figure 8.16). In this study, 38 fetuses were evaluated at 17–33 weeks of gestation. Of those, 18 were normal and 20 had trisomy 21. On 2D alone, 9/20 trisomy 21 fetuses had hypoplastic or absent nasal bones. However, using 3D and the x-ray mode, only three of those nine had true absence or hypoplasia of the nasal bone, since in those cases the abnormality involved one of the two nasal bones. Hence unilateral abnormalities of the fetal nasal bone were a new reported finding in trisomy 21, which, when present, may lead to misdiagnosis on 2D ultrasound. Benoit concluded that the maximal mode may aid in determining whether there is true hypoplasia or absence of the fetal nasal bone (Benoit and Chaoui 2005).

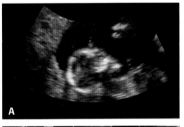
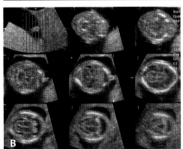
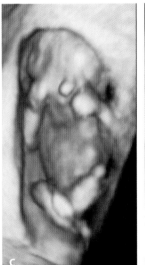
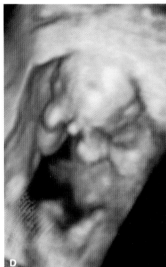

FIGURE 8.15 Fetus with proboscis examined at 12w6d and 14w6d. (A) Proboscis is suspected on 2D evaluation. (B) TUI of the fetal brain confirms abnormal intracranial anatomy with no "butterfly" created by the choroid plexus. (C, D) Fetus evaluated using surface rendering, clarifying the proboscis to the examiner as well as the family.

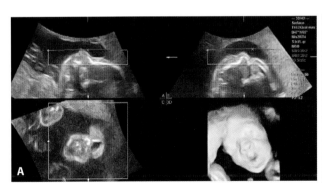
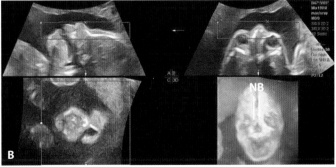

FIGURE 8.16 3D volume of a 22w6d fetus. (A) Volume displayed using surface rendering. (B) Subsequently, the volume is displayed in the maximum mode, clearly depicting both nasal bones (NB).

Subsequent to Benoit's study, Peralta et al. carried out a study on 450 fetuses in the first trimester to try to detect a gap between the two nasal bones in the first trimester (Peralta et al. 2005). In this study, a 3D volume was obtained at the time of the nuchal translucency assessment, which was analyzed using the multiplanar mode. Twenty percent of normal fetuses, were found to have a normal gap, a finding that may potentially lead to misdiagnosis of an absent nasal bone. In addition, with the lateral resolution of most machines approximately 0.6 mm, if the gap were to be greater than 0.6 mm, this could lead to the conclusion of an absent nasal bone.

MAXILLARY/MANDIBULAR ABNORMALITIES

The maxillary/mandibular area may be key in several dysmorphic syndromes (Figure 8.17). As a consequence, visualizing the fetal profile is of importance in all fetuses. However, obtaining the perfect mid-sagittal section is not always feasible. This is where volume sonography, with the ability to navigate through the volume, may be utilized.

In 2002 Lee et al. reported on nine cases of micrognathia in which 3D increased the chances of obtaining the true mid-sagittal section. In addition, surface rendering proved to be as useful as the multiplanar mode as an adjunct to the initial 2D image (Lee et al. 2002b).

> **CLINICAL UTILITY OF VOLUME SONOGRAPHY IN EVALUATING THE MAXILLA AND MANDIBLE**
>
> 1. Facilitates obtaining the true mid-sagittal section to assess the fetal profile
> 2. Facilitates the measurement of the maxillary and mandibular size

Dagklis et al. reported on the use of the 3D multiplanar mode for measuring the maxillary depth to detect midfacial hypoplasia in 862 normal fetuses and 80 trisomy 21 fetuses. They found that the maxillary depth is shorter in trisomy 21 fetuses (hence the flat face) by approximately 0.3 mm. The results of their study demonstrated that this measuement was not useful because the small difference between normal and abnormal fetuses was within the limits of the axial resolution of the sonographic machine (Dagklis et al. 2006). Subsequently, Roelfsema et al. used 3D to determine normograms for maxillary and mandibular size in 126 fetuses at 18–34 weeks, demonstrating that the measurement was more feasible when utilizing 3D rendering (Roelfsema et al. 2006).

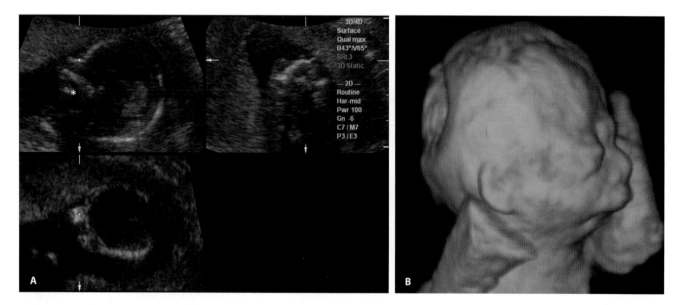

FIGURE 8.17   3D volume of a 22w0d fetus with microretrognathia is obtained. (A) Volume is displayed in the three orthogonal planes. Note the reference dot localizing the nasal bone in all three planes. Note the mandible (*) in plane A. (B) Volume is rendered using the surface mode, clearly depicting the microretrognathia.

Neck Abnormalities

One of the earliest reports on the use of volume sonography was describing facial tumors and differentiating a cystic hygroma from a thickened nuchal translucency (Figure 8.18 and 8.19). Bonilla-Musoles et al. rescanned 25 fetuses and used volume sonography to characterize their neck masses. Characteristics used were bullae as well as the extent, amplitude, and the lack of membrane regularity, to further define the malformation as a cystic hygroma or a nuchal translucency. It was concluded that 3D was helpful in 70% of the cases (Bonilla-Musoles et al. 1998).

> **CLINICAL UTILITY OF VOLUME SONOGRAPHY IN EVALUATING THE FETAL NECK**
>
> 1. Characterizing neck tumors and differentiating a cystic hygroma from a thick nuchal translucency
> 2. Proper sizing of fetal goiter and determining the extent of response to therapy

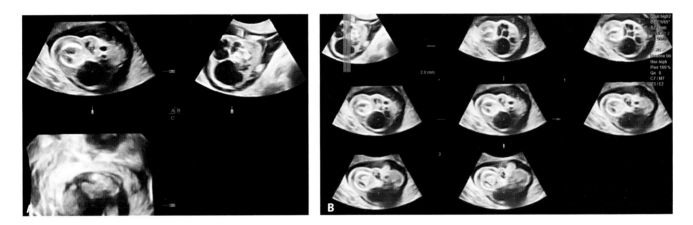

FIGURE 8.18 3D volume of a 16w5d fetus with a septated cystic hygroma. (A) Volume is displayed in the multiplanar mode. (B) Volume is displayed using TUI at an interslice thickness of 2 mm and VCI at a slice thickness of 2 mm, and using sepia as the color. The reference dot is placed in the largest cyst, localizing it in all eight panes.

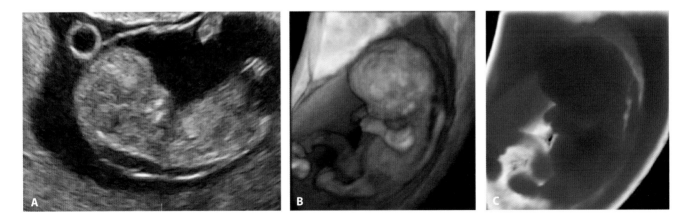

FIGURE 8.19 A transvaginally acquired volume of 9w3d fetus with a visible nuchal translucency. (A) Fetus in 2D showing the NT. (B) NT as seen utilizing surface rendering. (C) NT as seen using HD*live* render mode.

A fetal goiter was examined by 3D and power Doppler angiography by Nath et al. The true benefit was in following its volume and response to therapy, but most importantly, in aiding the parents to appreciate the goiter, and this proved to be the major incentive for their compliance (Nath et al. 2005).

OTHER USES OF VOLUME SONOGRAPHY IN EVALUATION OF THE FETAL FACE

Several other areas in the fetal face have been evaluated by volume sonography, as listed below.

OTHER USES FOR VOLUME SONOGRAPHY IN THE EVALUATION OF THE FETAL FACE

1. Ectodermal dysplasia
2. Congenital ichthyosis "Harlequin" fetus
3. Determining the in-utero craniofacial variability index (CVI)
4. Dysmorphologies: cebocephaly, trisomies, otocephaly, Treacher Collins, cat-eye syndrome

---

Several case reports have concluded that 3D is helpful in visualizing the details of the face, ears, and lips in confirming ectodermal dysplasia, trisomy 18, frontonasal malformations, cat-eye syndrome, cebocephaly, otocephaly, cases of unusual facial clefting, and Treacher Collins syndrome. The greatest benefit was in helping the parents appreciate the abnormality (Lin et al. 1998; Hsu et al. 2002; Shipp et al. 2002; Tanaka et al. 2002; Sepulveda et al. 2003; Volpe et al. 2004; Pilu et al. 2005; Allen and Maestri 2008; Allen et al. 2008; Zheng et al. 2008).

Another utility for volume sonography has been demonstrated by Benoit (1999), Bongain et al. (2002), and Vohra et al. (2003): the prenatal diagnosis of congenital ichthyosis, the "Harlequin" fetus. This is a rare congenital abnormality that cannot be diagnosed by 2D alone. Utilizing volume sonography enables confirmation of the typical "fish mouth" and fixed upper extremities.

In addition, and due to the complexity of the evaluation of the fetal face, Roelfsema et al. have developed a comprehensive detailed sonographic technique for establishing fetal craniofacial biometry. This craniofacial variability index (CVI) consists of 16 different measurements of the fetal face. For their evaluation, 136 normal fetuses and six abnormal fetuses were evaluated by volume sonography at 18–34 weeks of gestation. Anthropometry and cephalometry were utilized in establishing Z scores. The study concluded that when, in the absence of intrauterine growth retardation, two or more abnormal Z scores are present, this may be indicative of dysmorphology (Roelfsema et al. 2007a). In a subsequent study by the same group on seven syndromic fetuses and seven with isolated facial clefts, a higher CVI was found in the more severe bilateral clefts. In addition, CVI was higher and there were more abnormal Z scores in the syndromic fetuses versus those with isolated clefts. The conclusion was that this could be a differentiating method between syndromic fetuses and those with isolated facial clefts (Roelfsema et al. 2007b).

In summary, the fetal face, a most elusive, complex area of the fetus, can undergo extensive evaluation with the use of volume sonography. The key is to look beyond the "pretty face," become familiar with the complex techniques, and know when to employ them in order to differentiate syndromic cases from those with isolated abnormalities.

LIMITATIONS OF VOLUME SONOGRAPHY IN THE EVALUATION OF THE FETAL FACE

Though volume sonography certainly helps clarify several complicated facial abnormalities and may help provide more evidence to a potential underlying chromosomal aberration (Figure 8.20), it nonetheless may provide false reassurance. Caution must be exercised in cases of trisomies where a 3D-rendered image may be highly suggestive of a normal fetus with no discernable facial features to suggest a fetus affected by trisomy 21. This is precisely why the suspicion should rely on the well-established basic 2D sonographic markers. In addition, although volume sonography has been shown to be of value in certain cases of skin abnormalities such as in the "Harlequin" fetus (Bongain et al. 2002), it has not been shown to be of diagnostic value in cases of skin denudation syndromes (Abu-Rustum et al. 2013) (Figure 8.21).

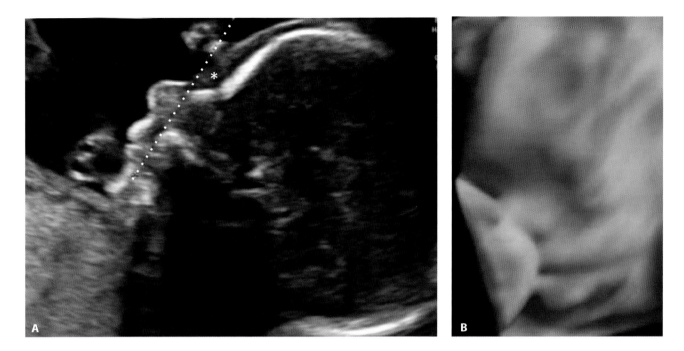

FIGURE 8.20 3D volume of a 21w2d fetus with suspected trisomy 21. (A) 2D image of the fetal profile with an abnormally close mandibular-maxillary line (dotted line) and prenasal thickness (*). (B) Volume displayed using HD*live* depicting the up-slanting palpebral fissures and small nose. This fetus was confirmed to have Down syndrome.

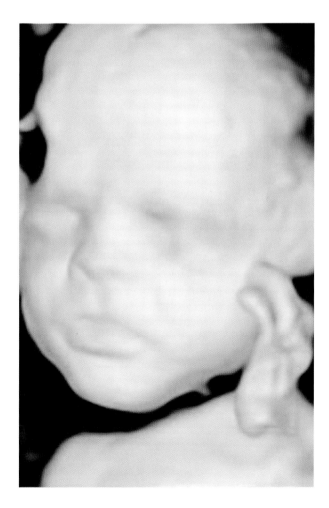

FIGURE 8.21 3D volume of a 33w2d fetus presenting with polyhydramnios, echogenic amniotic fluid, and echogenic debris within the stomach. Evaluation of the fetal face was falsely reassuring. The patient delivered on the same day of the scan and the newborn was found to be affected by epidermolysis bullosa with extensive facial involvement. Depiction of skin denudation is a major limitation of 3D ultrasound.

CONCLUSION

Volume sonography has an important role in the clarification of abnormalities involving the fetal face. It also has a great role in early reassurance, which may be possible from the first trimester, to ease the anxiety of families having prior affected offspring (Figure 8.22). The greatest benefit is in the extensive evaluation of facial clefts. Nonetheless, the techniques are complicated, require expertise, and one must keep in mind the various artifacts that may be introduced and that might ultimately lead to false diagnoses or reassurances. Therefore the user must be familiar with the available techniques and should gain expertise in utilizing them in normal fetuses in order to be able to properly utilize them in cases of a suspected abnormality. The gold standard remains a good 2D image. Any suspicion of a facial abnormality may be clarified further with the proper utilization of 3D sonography.

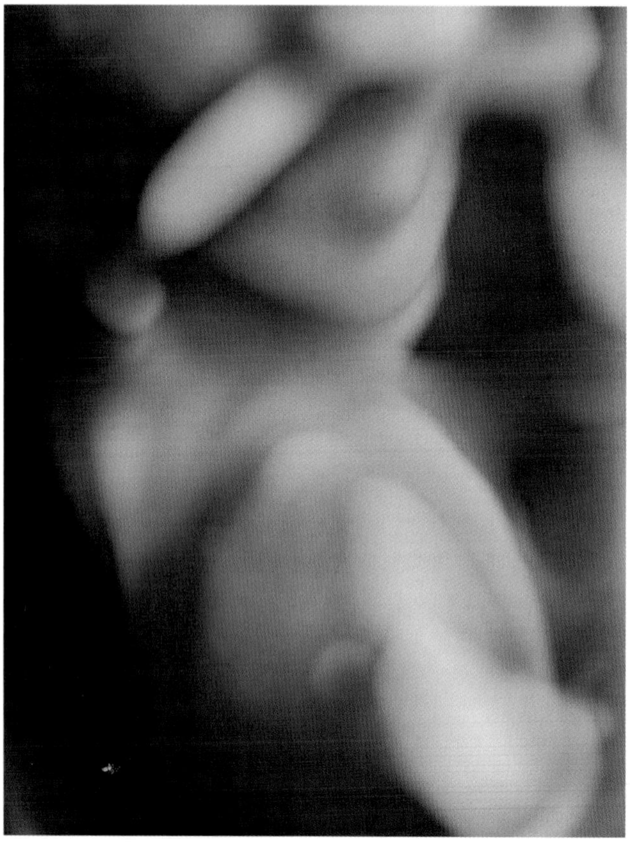

FIGURE 8.22 3D volume of the fetal face of a 12w3d fetus rendered using HD*live*, depicting an intact upper lip and providing invaluable early reassurance to a family with a prior affected child.

PRACTICAL PEARLS

- The key to a good 3D image is a good 2D image
- Attempt getting a volume with a good fluid interphase
- Avoid volumes with motion, a limb, the placenta, or cord in front of the fetal face
- When evaluating the fetal face, get a volume of the profile for a final en-face rendered image. You may also use VCI-C by putting the green line in front of the profile
- When evaluating the fetal face, get an en-face volume for a final rendered image of the profile. An oblique approach may even provide a better image and it requires less fluid as an interphase (Benoit oral communication 2012)
- For evaluation of the external surface, a lower quality for volume acquisition may be utilized as it may generate a smoother face (Benoit oral communication 2012)
- To generate a nice profile on a black background commence with an en-face fetal face, MagiCut the half of the face of lower quality then rotate the face by 90 degrees to depict the profile (Benoit oral communication 2012)
- To examine the fetal palate, use the maximum mode in the reverse-, flipped- or oblique-face techniques, or any combination of the above
- The OmniView algorithm enables the simultaneous display of 3 non-orthogonal planes of the face
- You may lower the gain for evaluating the face or decrease the gain while post-processing
- When rendering with HD*live*, adjusting the shadow softness leads to more natural images of the fetus (Benoit oral communication 2012)

9 Clinical Applicability in the Fetal Central Nervous System

INTRODUCTION

The brain is one of the most challenging areas to image in the fetus. This is due to the fact that for a full evaluation, several planes are required, and those planes are not parallel to each other. Some of these planes are oblique, making the evaluation difficult. In addition, there is the challenge of obtaining the mid-coronal plane, and this further limits a complete assessment. With the advent of volume sonography, visualizing all these planes can be facilitated if one were to obtain a 3D volume of the brain and then properly navigate through it, utilizing the various available tools and techniques.

CLINICAL UTILITY

Although a good 2D image remains the mainstay and the basis for a good 3D image, numerous studies have addressed the utility and advantages of volume sonography for the fetal central nervous system (CNS). The primary areas of interest that have demonstrated added benefit are those involving sonoembryology and characterizing normal development (discussed in Chapter 7), evaluating the cranial sutures (Figure 9.1), the corpus callosum (Figure 9.2), angiography of vascular malformations, as well as clarifying subtle differences, leading to more accurate diagnoses in CNS anomalies.

> ### UTILITY OF VOLUME SONOGRAPHY IN CNS EVALUATION
>
> 1. Sonoembryology
> 2. Skull
> 3. Cranial sutures
> 4. Corpus callosum
> 5. Vascular malformations
> 6. Other areas

SONOEMBRYOLOGY

Several authors have looked at the role of volume sonography in fetal development. One of the earliest studies was by Blaas et al. (1995) in which they were able to visualize structures of a few mm using 3D sonography. Viñals et al. used volume- contrast imaging (VCI) on 203 fetuses to establish normograms for the developing cerebellar vermis at 18–23 (Viñals et al. 2005). In 2007, Mittal et al. used volume sonography to look at the development of the sylvian fissure starting at 12 weeks. They were able to identify 99% of sylvian fissures from 12 weeks on (Mittal et al. 2007). Sepulveda et al. used 3D sonography to ascertain holoprosencephaly at 9w6d (Sepulveda et al. 2007) (Figure 9.3). Roelfsema et al. reported on the use of 3D for

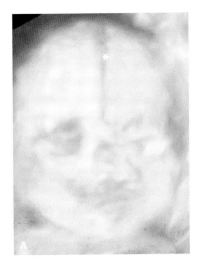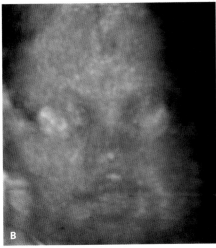

FIGURE 9.1 Metopic sutures. (A) Maximum mode is used to render the volume from a 24w2d fetus, clearly depicting the metopic suture (*). (B) Maximum mode is used to evaluate a 34w4d fetus with suspected craniocynostosis. Note the absence of a clearly visible metopic suture in contrast to the fetus on the left.

prenatal skull development (Roelfsema et al. 2007c). Kim et al. carried out a hallmark study on the development of the fetal ventricular system using the inversion mode and MagiCut in fetuses at 7–12 weeks (Kim et al. 2008). Most recently, Zalel et al. used VCI and TUI to assess the timing of the appearance of the cerebellar vermis, which was detected in 40% of fetuses at 18 weeks, 94% of fetuses at 22 weeks, and 100% of fetuses at 25%. Nonetheless, this technique was not very useful for other structures in the posterior fossa (Zalel et al. 2009).

CLINICAL UTILITY OF VOLUME SONOGRAPHY IN SONOEMBRYOLOGY

1. Confirming holoprosencephaly in the first trimester
2. Following the natural development of different areas of the brain
3. Determining the sensitivity of ultrasound at each gestational age for visualizing various intracranial structures

---

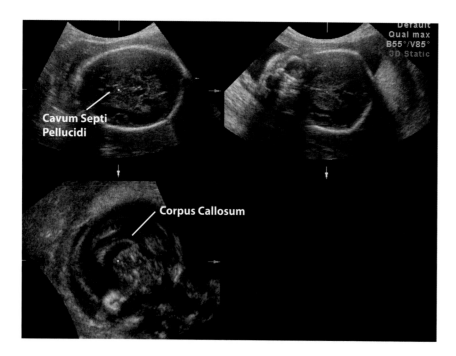

FIGURE 9.2 3D volume of a 22w6d fetus displayed in the multiplanar mode. The volume is acquired from the axial plane, plane A, automatically generating the plane of the corpus callosum in plane C.

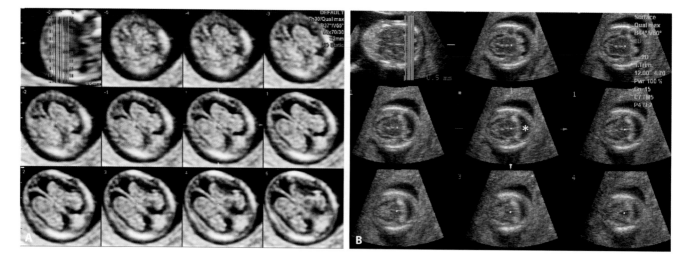

FIGURE 9.3 TUI of a normal and an abnormal brain. (A) TUI of a 12w5d normal fetal brain at an interslice thickness of 0.6 mm and a VCI thickness of 2 mm, depicting the "butterfly" formed by the choroid plexus filling the lateral ventricles. (B) TUI of a 12w6d abnormal fetal brain with holoprosencephaly at an interslice thickness of 0.6 mm and a VCI thickness of 2 mm. Note the absence of the butterfly, and the single ventricle (*).

THE SKULL

3D ultrasound helps clarify various anomalies of the bony skull, namely in cases of acrania and encephaloceles. Various modalities may be used, with the maximum mode being the most applicable, in order to show the bony defect. It is also possible to combine TUI with VCI in addition to surface rendering. Care must be taken in these cases, as the images generated may sometimes be quite unsettling for the family, and it is advisable to check with the family whether they prefer not to see any "colored" images. In such cases, off-line analysis may be carried out on stored volume data sets (Figures 9.4–9.6).

> ## CLINICAL UTILITY OF VOLUME SONOGRAPHY IN EVALUATING THE SKULL
>
> 1. Ascertains the intactness of the skull
> 2. Helps determine the extent of involvement of the brain and spine in case of a malformation
> 3. Clarifies the anomaly to the family

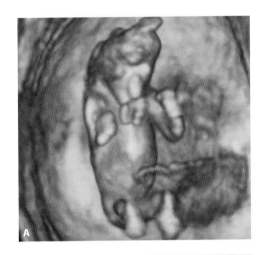
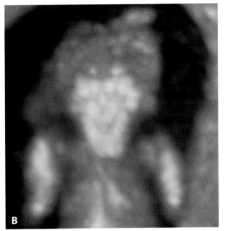

FIGURE 9.4 3D volumes of fetuses with acrania. (A) Surface-rendered 3D volume of a 12w0d fetus depicting protruding brain tissue and lack of bony structures above the orbits, consistent with acrania. (B) Another fetus with acrania at 13w3d. The volume is displayed using the maximum mode and showing absence of the skull.

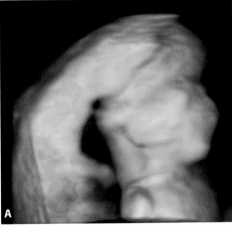
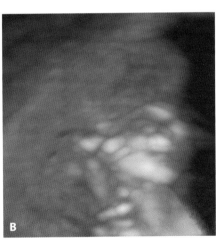

FIGURE 9.5 3D volume of a 12w0d fetus with acrania. (A) Volume is displayed using surface mode. (B) Volume is displayed using maximum mode confirming absence of the bony skull.

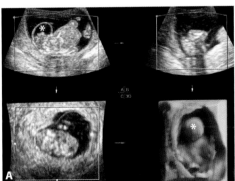
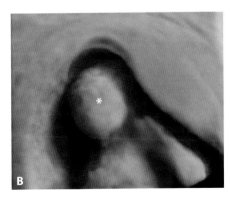

FIGURE 9.6 3D volume of a 15w3d fetus with a cystic structure posterior to the head. (A) Volume displayed in the multiplanar mode with surface rendering using HD*live*, confirming the presence of a posterior encephalocele. (B) Close up of the defect (*).

CRANIAL SUTURES

Abnormal development of the metopic sutures has been associated with several syndromes. However, visualizing these sutures (Table 9.1) and differentiating between molding and craniosynostosis has great limitations when 2D ultrasound is used. This is where 3D has had an invaluable role. Benacerraf et al. reported in 2000 on the role of 3D in arriving at a more definitive diagnosis of skull abnormalities, using 3D in a case of Pfeiffer syndrome at 26 weeks (Benacerraf et al. 2000). Another study was carried out by Krakow et al. in which 3D facilitated the visualization of the entire length of the suture lines, an otherwise impossible task, using 2D alone (Krakow et al. 2001). Dikkenboom et al. used 3D at 18–24 weeks to successfully visualize the cranial sutures in 82%–100% of cases. The sagittal and posterior sutures were seen in less than 50% of cases and the visualization was less accurate with advancing gestation (Dikkenboom et al. 2004). Faro et al. used surface and maximum modes to look at the process of ossification of the frontal bones and subsequent metopic suture development (Faro et al. 2005). Chaoui et al. (2005) characterized the abnormal development of the metopic sutures in various abnormalities that may lead to their premature closure, such as in cases of holoprosencephaly or in the case of corpus callosum abnormalities. Rochelson et al. carried this further, using geometric morphometric analysis

Table 9.1 Steps to Visualizing the Sutures

Step 1:	Obtain a volume of the mid-sagittal fetal face (Figure 9.7)
Step 2:	Render the volume using maximum mode (Figure 9.8)
Step 3:	Adjust the size of the render box with a primary focus on the metopic sutures (Figure 9.9)
Step 4:	Flip the rendered image by 180 degrees (Figure 9.10)
Step 5:	Select the single-pane view and rotate the volume along the X, Y and Z axes as needed to optimize the final rendered image (Figure 9.11)

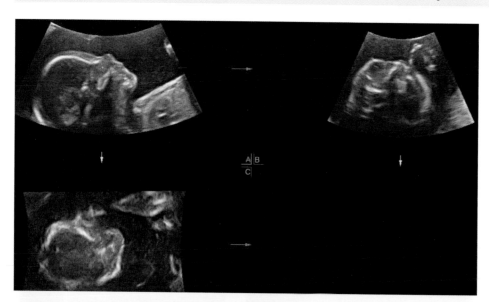

FIGURE 9.7 3D volume of a 21w2d fetus acquired starting from the sagittal plane and displayed in the multiplanar mode.

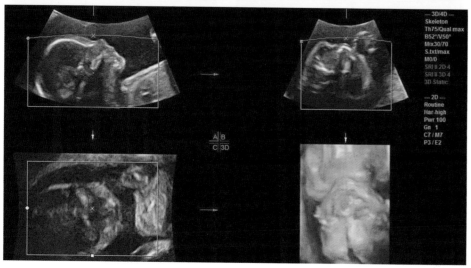

FIGURE 9.8 The same 3D volume of the 21w2d fetus in Figure 9.7 is subsequently displayed using the maximum mode.

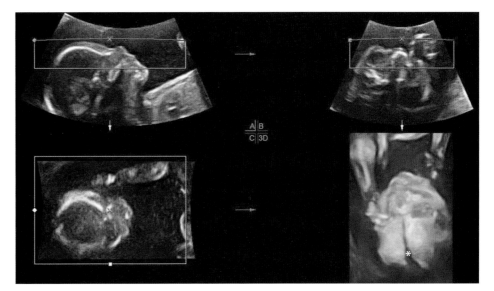

FIGURE 9.9 The same 3D volume of the 21w2d fetus in Figure 9.8 displayed in maximum mode. The size and location of the render box have been adjusted to focus on the metopic suture (*).

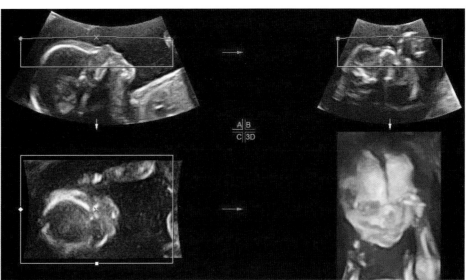

FIGURE 9.10 The final rendered image is now rotated by 180 degrees.

applied to 3D to quantify skull shape differences in normal and abnormal fetuses (Rochelson et al. 2006). In 2008, Fuchs et al. used translabial ultrasound to study the sutures and found VCI helpful in seeing details and the extent of rotation in labor (Viñals et al. 2005). Paladini et al. used VCI to examine the anterior fontanelle and found that it increases with advancing gestation but that its relative size to the volume of the fetal head decreases. It may be enlarged in fetuses with trisomy 21 (Paladini et al. 2007, 2008a).

CLINICAL UTILITY OF VOLUME SONOGRAPHY IN EVALUATING THE SUTURES

1. Differentiating molding from craniosynostosis
2. Visualizing the entire length of the suture line
3. Measuring the size of the anterior fontanelle

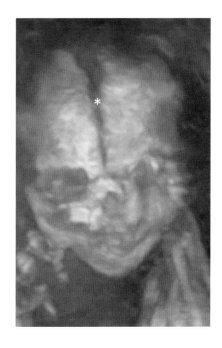

FIGURE 9.11 The single-pane view is selected to visualize the metopic suture (*) of the 21w2d fetus.

The Corpus Callosum

One of the biggest challenges in imaging the fetal brain is visualizing the corpus callosum, especially in cases of ventriculomegaly where it must be assessed to rule out agenesis of the corpus callosum (Figure 9.12 and 9.13). This is where volume sonography proves to be of benefit: through the use of the multiplanar mode with VCI (Table 9.2). As a result, various anomalies of the fetal brain (Figure 9.14 and 9.15), especially midline anomalies, are more easily visualized, enabling more accurate diagnosis of anomalies (Malinger et al. 2006). Timor-Tritsch reported that transvaginal transfontanelle 3D sonography is instrumental in diagnosing agenesis of the corpus callosum (Timor-Tritsch et al. 2000). Plasencia assessed the corpus callosum at 20–24 weeks and reported that the key is the angle of initial acquisition: if the acquisition is mid-sagittal, it has an echolucent appearance. If the acquisition is axial, it may appear echogenic (Plasencia et al. 2007).

> ### CLINICAL UTILITY OF VOLUME SONOGRAPHY IN VISUALIZING THE CORPUS CALLOSUM
>
> 1. Transvaginal transfontanelle view is extremely helpful
> 2. Multiplanar mode of properly acquired axial planes automatically generates corpus callosum views
> 3. Useful in ascertaining agenesis of the corpus callosum

Table 9.2 Steps to Visualizing the Corpus Callosum

Step 1:	Obtain a volume of the fetal head starting from the axial plane
Step 2:	Select the multiplanar mode and employ VCI (Figure 9.12A)
Step 3:	Plane (C) will automatically generate a display of the corpus callosum in the multiplanar mode (Figure 9.12A)
Step 4:	Select the single-pane view of plane C and magnify/crop as needed to optimize the final image of the corpus callosum (Figure 9.12B)

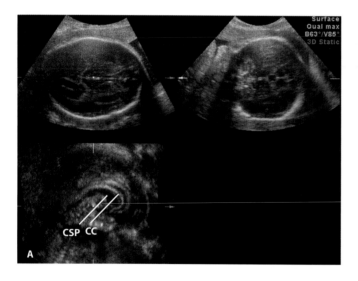
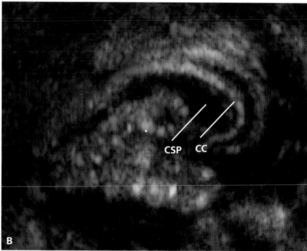

FIGURE 9.12   3D volume of a 27w1d fetus. (A) Volume acquired from the axial plane, plane A, and displayed in the multiplanar mode, automatically generating the sagittal plane in plane C. Plane C shows the corpus callosum (CC) and the cavum septi pellucidi (CSP). (B) Single-pane view is now selected, with a clearly visualized corpus callosum and cavum septi pellucidi. This is a difficult plane to obtain during routine scanning, and navigation through a properly acquired 3D volume facilitates ascertaining the presence of the corpus callosum.

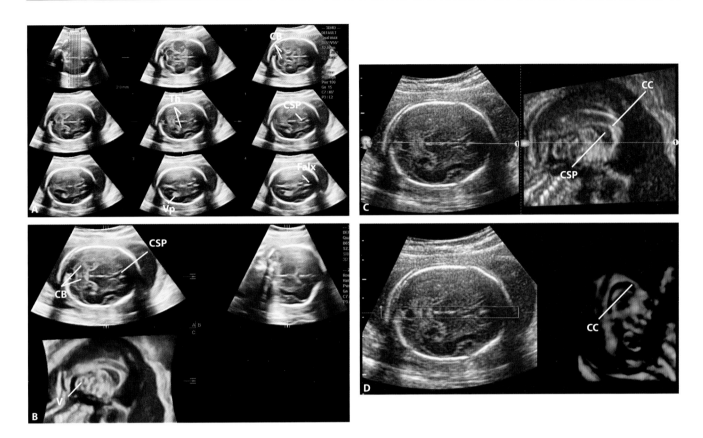

FIGURE 9.13 Accessing difficult planes in a 22w0d fetus. (A) Volume displayed in TUI at an interslice thickness of 2 mm and VCI with a slice thickness of 2 mm, showing the axial structures. (B) The same volume is now displayed using the multiplanar mode, automatically showing the challenging sagittal plane in plane C. (C) Using OmniView, the corpus callosum is seen. (D) Centering the render box over the midline generates a view of the corpus callosum using HD*live*. CB, cerebellum; Th, thalami; F, falx; CSP, cavum septi pellucidi; Vp, posterior horn of the lateral ventricle; V, vermis; CC, corpus callosum.

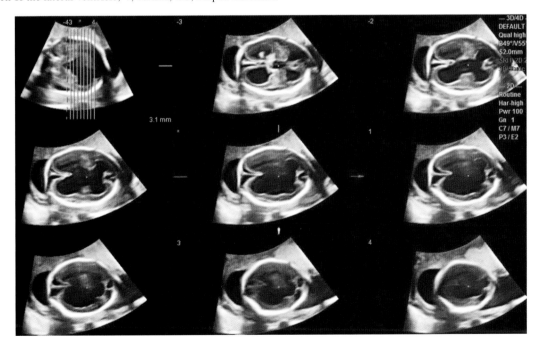

FIGURE 9.14 3D volume of a 19w4d fetus with hydranencephaly displayed using TUI at an interslice thickness of 3.1 mm and VCI at a slice thickness of 2 mm. Note the loss of normal architecture and the extent of involvement.

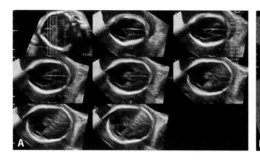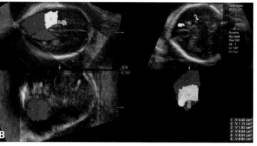

FIGURE 9.15 Volume of a 22w2d fetus with an encephalocele and a fluid-filled posterior fossa and complete distortion of the normal anatomy. (A) Volume displayed using TUI at an interslice thickness of 2 mm and VCI at a slice thickness of 2 mm. (B) The same volume is evaluated using SonoAVC general which automatically color codes the fluid-filled structures and calculates their volume for future monitoring.

VASCULAR MALFORMATIONS

One of the areas that has received great attention in the use of 3D ultrasound in the CNS has been 3D angiography for the visualization of the pericallosal vasculature (Figure 9.16) and the Circle of Willis (Table 9.3), and specifically in cases of vein of Galen malformations. Numerous case reports have proven the utility of 3D angiography in characterizing the aneurysmal malformation and its connections. Among the first was a case report by Lee on a fetus at 33 weeks with a cerebral cyst in which 3D assisted in diagnosing a vein of Galen aneurysm and precisely delineated the complicated vasculature. The conclusion was that this may provide guidance in postnatal management and may help predict prognosis more accurately (Lee et al.

2000). Bahlmann and Heling et al. reported on the use of 3D power angiography in the evaluation of an intracerebral cystic mass. It was found that the 3D power angiography results were comparable to MRI and that this technique had a significant impact on the diagnosis of fetal vascular anomalies (Bahlmann 2000; Heling et al. 2000). Ruano et al. reported on three fetuses and Gerards et al. reported on another two fetuses with vein of Galen malformations in which MRI was also used, and they found 3D power angiography helpful in visualizing the vascular malformations (Ruano et al. 2003a; Gerards et al. 2003). Gagel et al. used 3D power Doppler scanning and found it to be similar in accuracy to post-partum angiography in a vein of Galen malformation (Gagel et al. 2003). Most recently, Muench et al. reported on the use of 3D sonography and MRI in a fetal epidural hematoma (Muench et al. 2008).

Table 9.3 Steps to Visualizing the Circle of Willis

Step 1: Obtain a volume of the fetal head starting from the axial plane at the level of the thalami (Figure 9.17)
Step 2: Display the volume in the multiplanar mode (Figure 9.18)
Step 3: Render the volume with the glass-body mode (Figure 9.19)
Step 4: Select the single-pane view and optimize the final rendered image where minimum mode may be selected (Figure 9.20)
Step 5: Going back to step 3, another option is to display the volume using TUI (Figure 9.21)

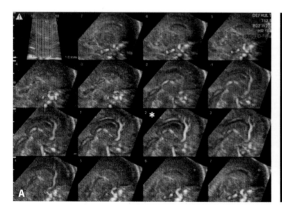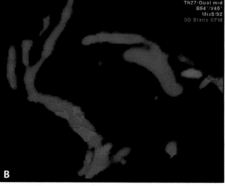

FIGURE 9.16 Imaging the pericallosal artery. (A) 3D STIC volume of a 21w6d fetus is acquired using HD-Flow. It is displayed using TUI at an interslice thickness of 1 mm, best depicting the pericallosal artery encircling the corpus callosum in the designated pane (*). This can be seen pulsating throughout a full cardiac cycle. (B) 3D volume of a 38w0d fetus with an intact corpus callosum and pericallosal artery as obtained using color Doppler and displayed using the minimum mode.

CLINICAL UTILITY OF VOLUME SONOGRAPHY IN VISUALIZING VASCULAR MALFORMATIONS

1. Visualizing vein of Galen aneurysm: characterizing the malformation and delineating the vascular connections
2. Detailed evaluation of cerebral vascular malformations
3. Evaluation of cerebral cystic masses

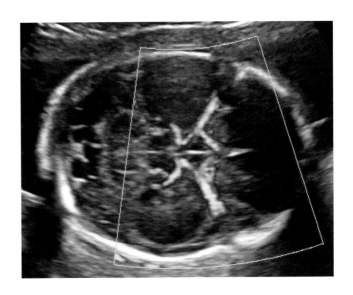

FIGURE 9.17 3D volume of a 24w3d fetus is obtained starting from the axial 2D plane (depicted here) at the level of the thalami. HD-Flow is utilized depicting the Circle of Willis.

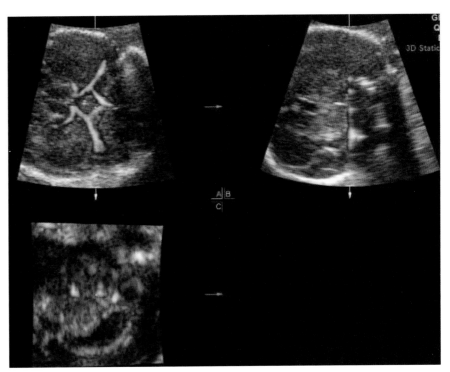

FIGURE 9.18 The same 3D volume in Figure 9.12 is now displayed in the multiplanar mode.

OTHER USES OF VOLUME SONOGRAPHY IN THE FETAL CNS

Several other areas involving the role of volume sonography in the fetal CNS have been studied. Those have involved midline structures, characterizing choroid plexus cysts (Figure 9.22) and the posterior fossa (Volpe et al. 2012) (Figure 9.23) as well as further assessing the presence of specific craniofacial abnormalities in particular syndromes. Timor-Tritsch et al. in 2000 used the transfontanelle 3D view and showed that it proved to be of great utility for review, consultation, and teaching (Timor-Tritsch et al. 2000). Paladini and Volpe used 3D to evaluate the posterior fossa and vermian morphometry in order to characterize vermian abnormalities (Paladini and Volpe 2006). Correa et al. found 3D neurosonography superior to 2D for visualizing the transcerebellar axial plane in 202 fetuses at 16–24 weeks (Correa et al. 2006; Varvarigos et al. 2002).

Pilu et al. found that although 2D had better quality in midline anomalies, 3D was easier and as effective for rapid assessment of the median plane of the head, and most useful when 2D proved to be difficult. The main downfall was evaluating the brainstem in this study (Pilu et al. 2006). Soto et al. used 3D as an adjunct to 2D to look at the skull mineralization in the absence of the occiput (Soto et al. 2006). Bault used 3D sonography to examine the optic chiasm (Bault 2006). Sepulveda used 3D reconstruction of the fetal skull and face to characterize the "helmet sign" of the forehead of a fetus with Wolf-Hirschhorn syndrome (Sepulveda 2007).

Viñals used the transfrontal 3D approach for assessing the midline structures. Though the overall 2D image was clearer, TUI proved to be helpful (Viñals et al. 2007; Ruano et al. 2004; Jouannic et al. 2005). In 2008, Levaillant and Mabille found 3D sonography easier than computed tomography (CT) and just as helpful in evaluating the sphenoid bone (Levaillant and Mabille 2005). Finally, in 2009, Benavides-Serralde et al. used volume sonography to assess the volume of intracranial structures in fetuses with intrauterine growth restriction. They found that all net volumes, primarily of the frontal areas, and with the exception of the thalamus, were smaller. They concluded that this might be attributable to neural reorganization in response to hypoxia (Benavides-Serralde et al. 2009).

CLINICAL UTILITY OF VOLUME SONOGRAPHY IN OTHER AREAS OF THE FETAL CNS

1. Useful for reviewing, teaching, and enabling off-line consultation
2. Useful in assessing skull mineralization
3. Enables examination of midline structures and the optic chiasm
4. May have a role in calculating the volume of intracranial structures in IUGR

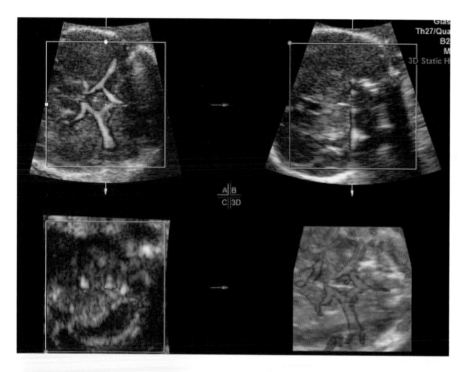

FIGURE 9.19 Volume is rendered using the glass-body mode that minimizes the gray-scale structures and highlights the vasculature.

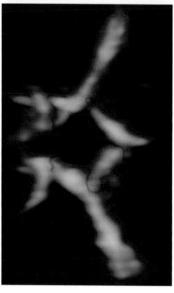

FIGURE 9.20 The size of the render box is now adjusted and enlarged to encompass the entire Circle of Willis. Minimum mode is selected which removes all gray-scale structures completely and clearly depicts the vasculature.

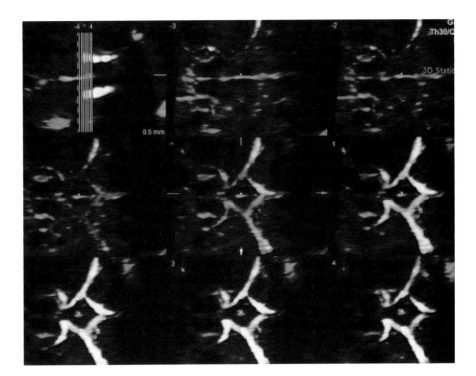

FIGURE 9.21 Another option is to display the volume after optimization, using TUI. In this image, the TUI interslice thickness is 0.5 mm and the VCI slice thickness is 2 mm

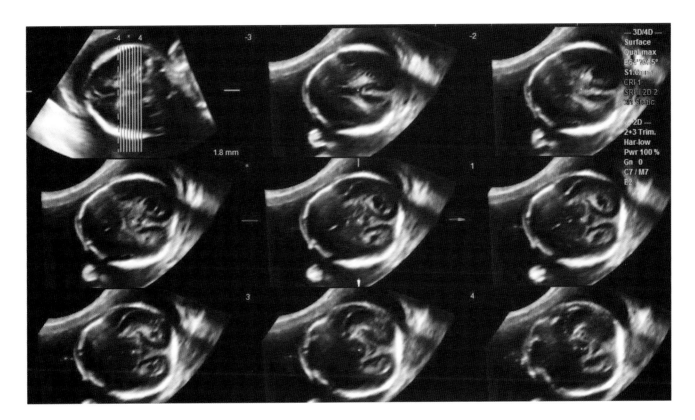

FIGURE 9.22 3D volume of a 21w0d fetus with brachycephaly and bilateral choroid plexus cysts displayed using TUI at an interslice distance of 1.8 mm and a VCI slice thickness of 1 mm.

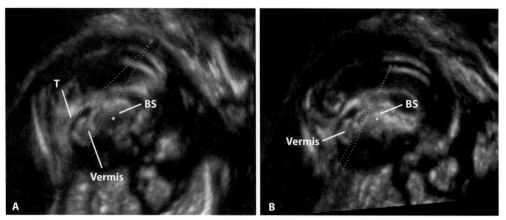

FIGURE 9.23 3D volume of the brain of a 22w6d fetus. (A) Navigating through the volume it is possible to generate the plane in which the brainstem–tentorium angle is measured. (B) Navigating through the volume, it is possible to generate the plane in which the brainstem–vermis angle is measured. This enables assessment of the posterior fossa for any abnormalities. BS: brain stem; T: tentorium.

LIMITATIONS OF VOLUME SONOGRAPHY IN EVALUATION OF THE FETAL CNS

The major limitation to utilizing 3D ultrasound for the fetal CNS is bone shadowing, especially with advancing gestation. This is where the transfontanelle approach, when feasible, proves to be of value in order to minimize the shadowing and resulting artifacts. Using 3D ultrasound in the study of the fetal brain is further complicated by the changing anatomy with advancing gestation in addition to the complex anomalies that distort most major anatomical landmarks. The study of the vasculature is quite challenging, and often times using HD-Flow rather than color Doppler may be helpful.

CONCLUSION

Volume sonography in the fetal CNS provides access to hard-to-reach central structures such as the corpus callosum, and structures in the posterior fossa such as the vermis. It also allows detailed study of the vasculature and is useful for reviewing, teaching, and off-line consultation. The quality of the underlying 2D image remains the key to a successful 3D image. Combining TUI with VCI results in marked improvement in the quality of the images. As such, learning how to properly utilize the various 3D techniques and modalities is invaluable in the evaluation of the fetal brain.

PRACTICAL PEARLS

- Whenever a skull defect is suspected, the maximum mode aids in ascertaining the presence of acrania
- A good acquisition of the fetal brain may be obtained through the transfontanelle window
- Starting with an axial plane, the multiplanar mode will automatically show the corpus callosum in plane C
- To avoid bone shadowing when acquiring a volume of the fetal brain, apply gentle pressure with a steady hand (Paladini oral communication 2013)
- An angle of 35-40 degrees is suitable for acquiring a volume of a second-trimester fetal brain
- A great advantage to displaying a volume of the fetal brain in the multiplanar mode is the ability to study the axial and sagittal planes simultaneously (Pilu oral communication 2013)

- For the evaluation of the posterior fossa and brainstem, it is helpful to acquire a volume starting with an axial plane in which both the cerebellum and cavum septi pellucidi are seen (Chaoui oral communication 2013)
- Utilizing VCI and TUI is instrumental to high-quality sectional analysis of the brain along any of the 3 axes
- Using VCI at a thickness of 2 mm together with the transparent mode allows optimal visualization of the cerebellum (Chaoui oral communication 2013)
- Properly utilizing 3D ultrasound in the evaluation of the fetal brain provides access to challenging structures and planes, is a great teaching tool and enables off-line consultation

10 Clinical Applicability in the Fetal Skeleton

INTRODUCTION

Various areas of the fetal skeletal system may be affected in several syndromes. For this reason, proper diagnosis of limb, thoracic, and skeletal dysplasias can be key in reaching the proper diagnosis. This ensures appropriate parental counseling for the current and future pregnancies. However, this evaluation is limited by the 2D approach used, and it may be enhanced through the utilization of volume sonography.

CLINICAL UTILITY

Numerous studies have been published over the years evaluating the use of volume sonography in the evaluation of the fetal skeleton. Although evidence for the diagnostic capabilities of volume sonography improving clinical management has not been marked, there has been a general consensus that it is helpful in further characterizing defects and clarifying diagnoses to the family as well as the medical team.

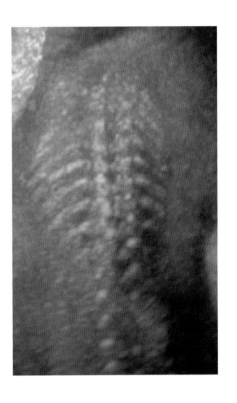

FIGURE 10.1 A 3D volume of a 23w3d fetus with Goldenhar syndrome displayed using maximum mode. Note the shortened, curved ribs.

AREAS IN WHICH VOLUME SONOGRAPHY MAY BE OF UTILITY

1. Rib cage
2. Spine
3. Limbs
4. Skeletal dysplasias
5. Iliac angle

Rib Cage

Although it is not routine practice to count the fetal ribs, this may be of use in certain syndromes. This task is almost impossible by 2D ultrasound but has been made possible with the availability of volume sonography. Assessing the number and presence of hemi vertebrae (Figure 10.1) as well as abnormal spacing between the ribs may be of diagnostic value. In 2002 Viora et al. reported that 3D sonography helped narrow the differential diagnosis in a fetus with short rib polydactyly (Viora et al. 2002). Sallout et al. reported that 3D sonography was complementary to 2D scanning once post-processing was utilized to enhance the image (Sallout et al. 2006). Gindes et al. reported on the utility of 3D ultrasound in counting the ribs of 75 fetuses and hinted at the possible association between an abnormal number of ribs (Figure 10.2) and childhood

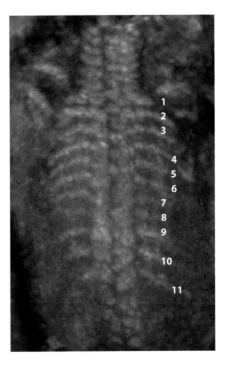
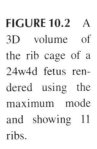

FIGURE 10.2 A 3D volume of the rib cage of a 24w4d fetus rendered using the maximum mode and showing 11 ribs.

malignancies (Gindes et al. 2008). Most recently, Izquierdo et al. reported on the utility of 3D sonography in describing the degree of extension of a cleft sternum (Izquierdo et al. 2009). Table 10.1 provides details on how to visualize the ribs.

CLINICAL UTILITY OF VOLUME SONOGRAPHY IN ASSESSING THE RIB CAGE

1. Counting the ribs
2. Ascertaining the presence of hemivertebrae

Table 10.1 **Steps to Visualizing and Counting the Ribs**

Step 1:	Start with a fetus in a sagittal lie, preferably in a spine-up position (Figure 10.3)
Step 2:	Obtain a 3D sweep (Figure 10.3)
Step 3:	Activate OmniView and rotate the render line to overlie the spine at the level of the rib cage with a slice thickness of 20 mm (Figure 10.4)
Step 4:	Select the single-pane view for an optimal depiction of the rib cage (Figure 10.5)

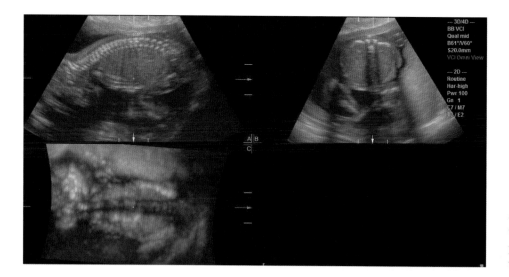

FIGURE 10.3 A 3D volume of a 21w4d fetus in a spine-up position is acquired from the sagittal plane. The volume is displayed in the multiplanar mode.

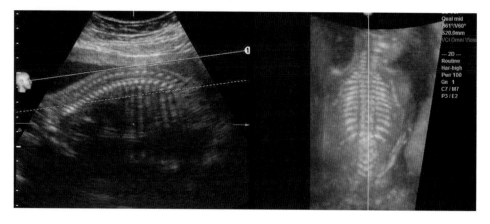

FIGURE 10.4 OmniView is activated with a VCI slice thickness of 20 mm and maximum mode display in order to generate an image of the fetal rib cage.

THE FETAL SPINE

The value of volume sonography in studying the fetal spine has been primarily evaluated with respect to development of the spine and localization of neural tube defects. There have been many methods utilized to display the fetal spine. OmniView, as with the rib cage, utilizes the reference dot for navigation within a volume, and images rendered in maximum mode. Table 10.2 describes a traditional multiplanar method for viewing the spine. Proper localization of the level of the defect in spina bifida is of utmost importance when it comes to counseling the family in regards to fetal prognosis. Schild et al. used 3D sonography in 103 women to study the developmental volume changes of the thoracolumbar spine between 16 and 25 weeks (Schild et al. 1999). Blaas et al. evaluated three fetuses with spina bifida prior to 10 weeks and found that 3D was not of much added value in detecting early spina bifida (Blaas et al. 2000a). Lee et al. found that 3D multiplanar views were complementary to 2D in localizing the defect, and were more informative than the rendered views (Figure 10.10 and 10.11) (Lee et al. 2002a).

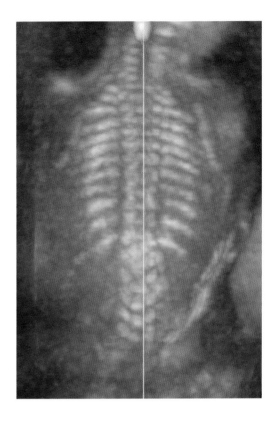

CLINICAL UTILITY OF VOLUME SONOGRAPHY IN ASSESSING THE FETAL SPINE

1. Enables evaluating the development of the spine
2. Facilitates localizing the level of the lesion in spina bifida

FIGURE 10.5 The single-pane view is subsequently selected. Note that the cervical, thoracic, and part of the lumbar spine is visible.

Table 10.2 **Steps to Visualizing the Fetal Spine**

Step 1:	Start with a fetus in a sagittal lie, preferably in a spine-up position; obtain a 3D volume and display it in the multiplanar mode (Figure 10.6)
Step 2:	Select the maximum mode and render the volume (Figure 10.7)
Step 3:	Adjust the size of the render box to optimize the rendered image with inclusion of the lumbosacral area (Figure 10.8)
Step 4:	Select the single-pane, rotate by 90 degrees, and adjust the color for an optimal depiction of the spine (Figure 10.9)

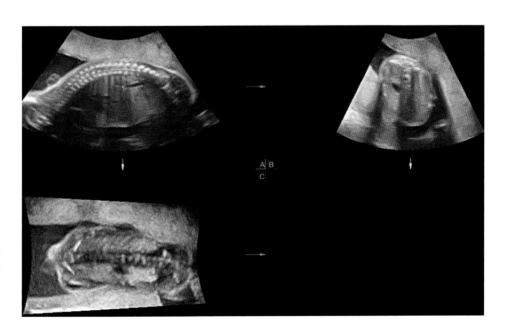

FIGURE 10.6 A 3D volume of a 21w6d fetus is obtained, starting with the sagittal spine-up position, and is displayed in the multiplanar mode.

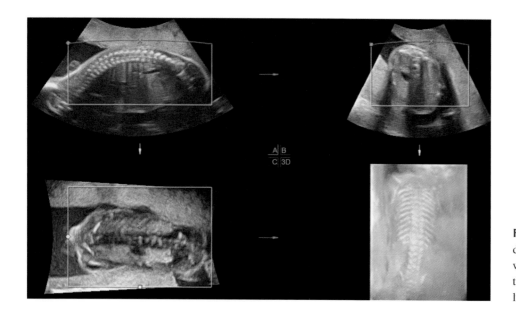

FIGURE 10.7 Volume is rendered using the maximum mode, with the render box covering the entire spine down to the lumbosacral region.

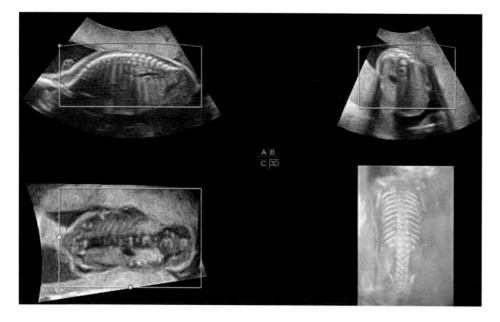

FIGURE 10.8 The rendered image is rotated and the threshold is adjusted.

LIMBS

One of the parents' first questions is always whether their fetus has all 10 fingers and toes. Although digit ascertainment using 2D ultrasound is useful, it is much clearer using 3D ultrasound where it is possible to manipulate the limbs and access them from various angles. This tends to be time consuming and is not recommended as part of routine screening, but is of diagnostic value in certain syndromes (Benacerraf 2008). One of the earliest studies was by Lee et al. on phocomelia where 3D was found to be of help to the parents (Lee et al 1995). Another study of normal and abnormal limbs was reported by Budorick et al. in 1998 in which they found that the limitations of 3D volumes were the same as in 2D sonography; however, there was

improved ability in the visualization of the limbs utilizing the multiplanar mode with volume rotation (Budorick et al. 1998) (Figure 10.12). Hata et al. carried out a prospective study on 77 fetuses across the gestations. They used surface rendering and not the multiplanar mode. They found surface rendering to be supplementary to 2D, especially with respect to enhancing the ability to visualize toes and fingers (Hata et al. 1998b). Several studies have also demonstrated that 3D sonography helped confirm the diagnosis of sirenomelia (Figure 10.13) and enabled the parents to visualize the abnormality. In addition, 4D assisted in determining the extent of movement or lack thereof (Monteagudo et al. 2002; Blaicher et al. 2001) (Figure 10.14). Hull et al. studied the presence of artifacts while visualizing the lower extremities and concluded that there were more artifacts

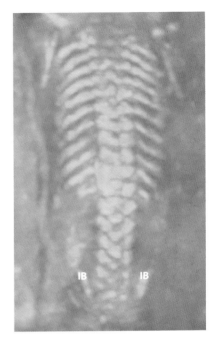

FIGURE 10.9 The single-pane view is selected and the render color is changed, enabling evaluation of the lumbosacral spine with the iliac bones (IB) visible on either side.

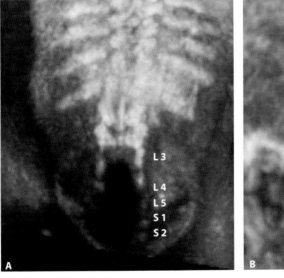

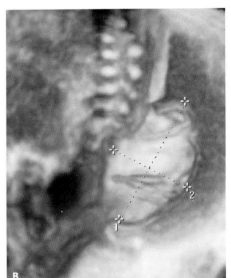

FIGURE 10.10 A 3D volume of a 26w2d fetus with spina bifida. (A) Volume is displayed using the maximum mode in an attempt to localize the level of the lesion. (B) Using surface rendering, the meningomyelocele is displayed and the anomaly is clarified to the family.

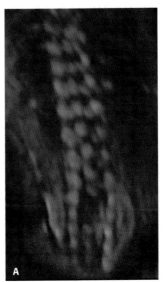

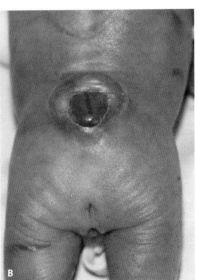

FIGURE 10.11 A 3D volume of a 20w5d fetus with spina bifida. (A) Volume is displayed using the maximum mode, depicting the lumbosacral involvement. (B) Neonate at birth.

while visualizing the lower limbs in comparison to the upper limbs due to flexion of the upper limbs (Hull et al. 2000). In addition, 3D is helpful in ascertaining the presence of an abnormal number of digits (Figure 10.15), or club feet (Figure 10.16).

CLINICAL UTILITY OF VOLUME SONOGRAPHY IN ASSESSING THE FETAL LIMBS

1. Facilitates counting the digits
2. Clarifies the appearance of sirenomelia to the parents
3. Helps in ascertaining limb abnormalities

SKELETAL DYSPLASIAS

Skeletal dysplasias (Figure 10.17) cover a wide spectrum of syndromes, with subtle differences involving various areas, and varying degrees of bone ossification. Moeglin et al. evaluated the role of surface rendering in two cases of achondroplasia and concluded that it allowed sequential and systemic visualization of the fetal skull, rachis, thorax, pelvis, long bones, and extremities (Moeglin et al. 2001). Ruano et al. used both surface and skeletal modes as well as 4D in the diagnosis of three cases of fetal akinesia deformation sequence. It was the 4D imaging that was of most help to the parents in understanding the fixed problem and its severity (Ruano et al. 2003a). In studying five cases of prenatal onset of skeletal dysplasia, Krakow et al. found that 3D

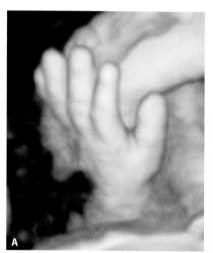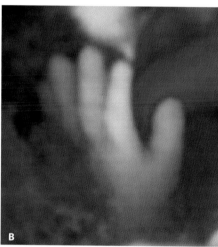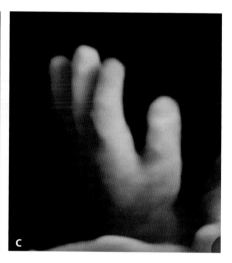

FIGURE 10.12   Volume of the hand and digits of a 27w0d fetus displayed using three modalities: (A) surface rendering, (B) dynamic rendering, and (C) HD*live*.

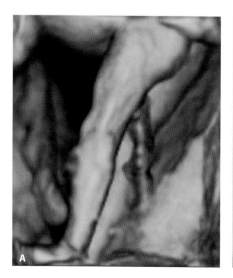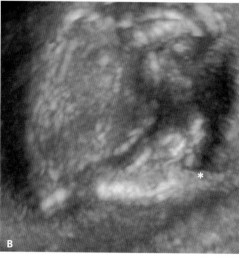

FIGURE 10.13   The lower limbs as examined using 3D ultrasound. (A) Buttocks and legs of a normal 21w3d fetus. (B) Volume of a 14w6d fetus with sirenomelia rendered using maximum mode, displaying a single wide lower extremity with abnormal ossification in the distal portion (*).

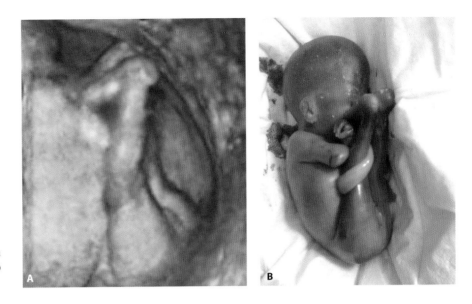

FIGURE 10.14 A 22w6d fetus with arthrogryposis. (A) Evaluated using 3D surface rendering. (B) Postmortem.

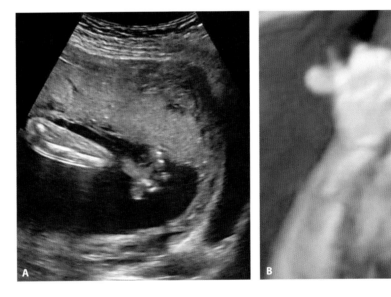

FIGURE 10.15 An evaluation of the hand of a 22w2d fetus. (A) 2D image raising suspicion for polydactyly. (B) 3D volume rendered using dynamic rendering, clearly showing the postaxial polydactyly.

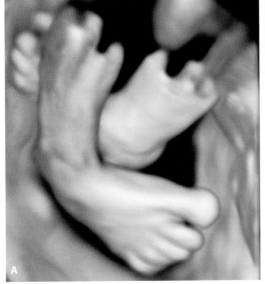
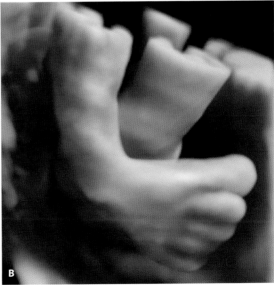

FIGURE 10.16 A 3D volume of a 27w4d fetus with bilateral club feet displayed using (A) Surface rendering and (B) HD*live*.

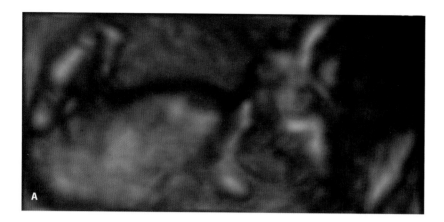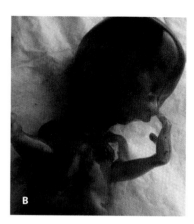

FIGURE 10.17   A 12w6d fetus with multiple anomalies. (A) 3D volume using surface rendering depicting rhizomelia with proximal short-ening of the humerus and femur. (B) Postnatal image confirming the findings (postnatal image courtesy of Adba Frangieh, MD).

was helpful primarily in the face and limbs and in assessing the relative proportion of the appendicular skeletal system as well as improving visualization to confirm the suspected diagnosis (Krakow et al. 2003). Sepulveda et al. reported on a more clear image with 3D in a case of diastrophic dys-plasia, specifically in visualizing the "hitchhiker's thumbs" (Sepulveda 2004). Ruano et al. evaluated the role of 3D and 3D helical tomography in six cases of skeletal dysplasias and found them to be complementary to 2D and useful (Ruano 2004c). Another report on ecterodactyly-ectodermal-dys-plasia by Allen et al. concluded that 3D was not essential but was helpful especially to the parents (Allen et al. 2008).

> **CLINICAL UTILITY OF VOLUME SONOGRAPGHY IN EVALUATING SKELETAL DYSPLASIAS**
>
> 1. Useful in assessing bone ossification
> 2. Aids in the systemic evaluation of the skull, rachis, thorax, pelvis, long bones, and extremities
> 3. Allows visualizing movement limitations in specific disorders

Iliac Angle

The iliac angle is reportedly wider in fetuses with trisomy 21, but is difficult to measure. For this reason, Lee et al. evaluated the role of 3D in an attempt to standardize its measurement in 35 normal fetuses and 16 trisomy 21 fetuses. It was concluded that standardization was possible in the axial plane but was found to be unreliable in the coronal plane (Lee et al. 2001).

> **CLINICAL UTILITY OF VOLUME SONOGRAPHY IN MEASURING THE ILIAC ANGLE**
>
> 1. Allows the standardization of measuring the iliac angle in the axial plane

Sacrococcygeal Teratoma

Two studies have looked at the role of 3D in the prenatal diag-nosis of sacrococcygeal teratomas. The first was by Bonilla-Musoles et al. in 2002 on two fetuses where it was found that with 3D there is the ability to rotate the image and remove obscuring items, enabling determination of the degree of sacral involvement and the extent of involvement of other pel-vic organs (Bonilla-Musoles et al. 2002). Another study by Roman et al. on a first-trimester fetus with a sacrococcygeal teratoma found 3D to be of most value in counseling the fam-ily and enabling them to visualize the abnormality (Roman et al. 2004).

> **CLINICAL UTILITY OF VOLUME SONOGRAPHY IN EVALUATING SACROCOCCYGEAL TERATOMAS**
>
> 1. Helps in determining the extent of sacral involvement
> 2. Clarifies the abnormality to the family, especially in the first trimester

LIMITATIONS OF VOLUME SONOGRAPHY IN EVALUATION OF THE FETAL SPINE

As with the various organ systems covered thus far, volume sonographic techniques require skill and training. In addition, in the presence of an anomaly, it becomes more challenging to acquire the optimal volume and render it to satisfaction.

CONCLUSION

Two areas where 3D ultrasound has been shown to be of clinical utility with respect to the fetal skeleton are counting the ribs and determining the level of involvement in the case of a neural tube defect, otherwise not possible with routine 2D sonography. In addition, 3D ultrasound is of value in evaluating the various components of the fetal skeleton and clarifying the findings to the family as early as the first trimester (Figure 10.18). And as with other areas of the fetus, this requires practice, skill, and an optimal basic 2D image from which to acquire the 3D volume.

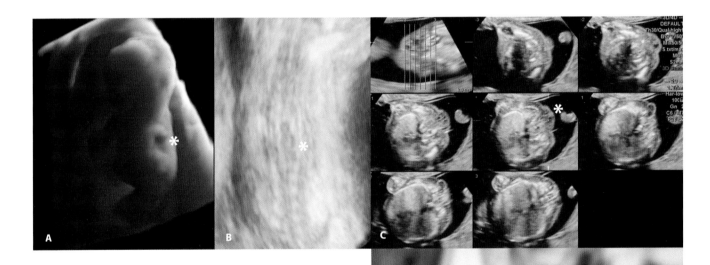

FIGURE 10.18   A 3D volume of a 12w6d fetus with spina bifida (*). The 3D images helped clarify the anomaly to the family given the extremely early gestational age. (A) The volume is rendered using HD*live* clearly illustrating the defect. (B) The volume is rendered using the skeleton mode depicting the bony defect. (C) The volume is rendered with TUI at an interslice distance of 2 mm and VCI at a slice distance of 2 mm depicting the extent of the defect. Note the reference dot localizing the defect. (D) The volume is rendered using OmniView with VCI at a slice thickness of 1 mm where the threshold and mix have been adjusted to generate this image.

PRACTICAL PEARLS

- Obtain multiple volumes of an anomaly
- VCI and OmniView are most helpful in evaluating the fetal spine
- OmniView, using the nonlinear option, allows tracing along the curvature of the spine for optimal visualization particularly if the fetus is flexed
- OmniView using two properly placed lines on either side of the spine allows thorough study of the fetal spine
- Always evaluate the spine with various modalities: maximum mode, OmniView, surface mode, etc.
- Remember to thoroughly evaluate the spine all the way down to the sacrum in order to exclude sacral agenesis

11 Clinical Applicability in the Fetal Cardiovascular System

INTRODUCTION

One of the most complex structures, and one that has eluded sonographers for years, is the fetal heart. This is a result of several factors, mainly its size and the challenges of studying a tiny beating organ in a moving fetus through the maternal abdomen. In addition, the fetal heart is the one organ whose appearance changes with the cardiac cycle; the sonographer must be aware of where in the cardiac cycle certain views are obtained for optimal interpretation and diagnosis. Despite the technological advances and the sophisticated machines we now have, congenital heart disease, which affects 8.8/1000 live births (Hoffman et al. 1978), is still suboptimally diagnosed prenatally, even in the best of hands, with recent reports of 57% detection from tertiary care centers (Tegnander et al. 2006). However, proper training and a systematic approach have been shown to translate into improved prenatal detection rates (Hunter et al. 2000). Early detection has been proven to be of great value, not only for preparing the family, but also for a timely delivery at a tertiary care center for optimal management of the newborn. With the advent of volume sonography, it is now possible to obtain off-line analysis and consultation from anyone with internet access, irrespective of where they are geographically. In addition, with the introduction of automation, standardization of fetal volumes for computer-aided analysis is now possible in order to improve our detection rates (Abuhamad et al. 2004, 2005, 2006, 2007).

CLINICAL UTILITY

Utilizing volume sonography, the fetal heart may be evaluated in any of several modalities in which B-Flow (Figure 11.1), color (Figure 11.2) and power Doppler (Figure 11.3), HD-Flow (Figure 11.4), and inversion mode (discussed in Chapter 5, Table 5.1, Figures 5.10–5.15) may be employed (Figure 11.5 and 11.6). Using these modalities, thorough assessment of the fetal heart is possible in order to improve the diagnosis of congenital cardiac defects. In fetal echocardiography, the volume can be displayed in any of several ways, as listed below.

TECHNIQUES THAT MAY BE UTILIZED FOR THE EVALUATION OF THE FETAL HEART

1. Standard 3D static (Figure 11.7)
2. Rendered 3D static (Figure 11.8)
3. STIC (Figure 11.9)
4. VCAD (Figures 11.10–11.20)

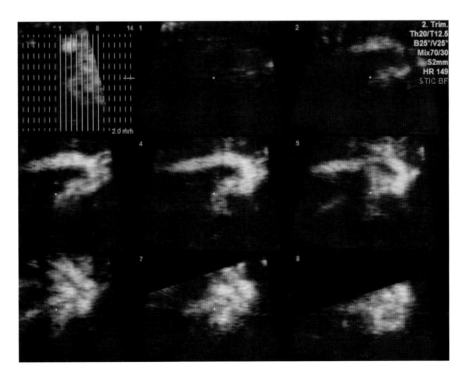

FIGURE 11.1 A STIC volume of a 21w4d aortic arch displayed utilizing B-Flow in TUI with an interslice thickness of 2 mm and VCI with a slice thickness of 2 mm. This generates an image akin to that obtained utilizing angiography.

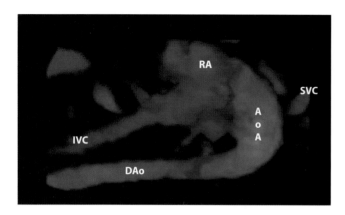

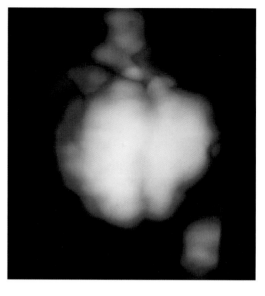

FIGURE 11.2 A 3D volume of the right atrial inflow, aortic arch and descending aorta of a 22w0d fetus. The volume was acquired using color Doppler in the minimum mode, hence creating a vascular cast. RA, right atrium; SVC, superior vena cava; IVC, inferior vena cava; AoA, aortic arch; DAo, descending aorta.

FIGURE 11.4 A STIC volume of a 13w3d fetal heart with HD-Flow. The volume is rendered in the minimum mode creating a cast of the heart that can be rotated along any of the *X, Y,* and *Z* axes. The symmetry of the chambers is illustrated.

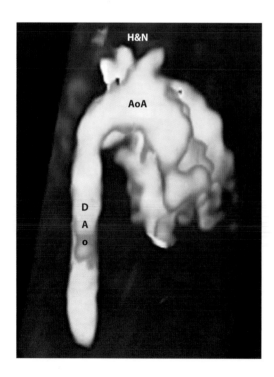

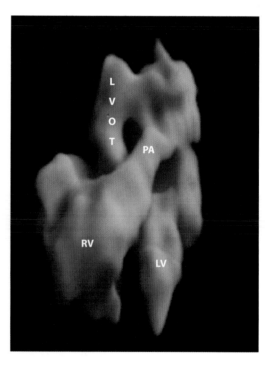

FIGURE 11.3 A 3D volume of the aortic arch and descending aorta of a 23w1d fetus. The volume was acquired using power Doppler in the minimum mode, hence creating a vascular cast. The aortic arch, head and neck vessels, and descending aorta are clearly depicted. The final rendered image is reassuring against the presence of an aortic coarctation. AoA, aortic arch; DAo, descending aorta; H&N, head and neck vessels.

FIGURE 11.5 A STIC volume of the fetal heart and aortic arch at 23w0d rendered using the inversion mode and HD*live*, depicting the right and left ventricles (RV, LV) and outflow tracts. PA, pulmonary artery; LVOT, aorta.

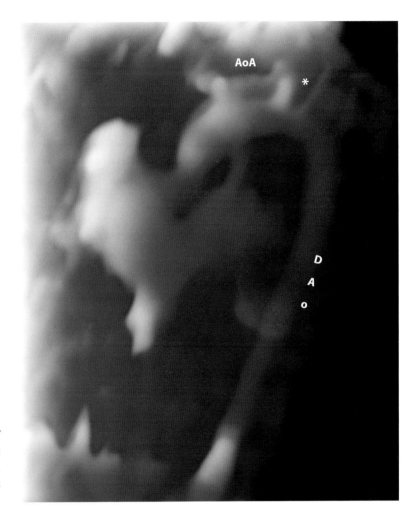

FIGURE 11.6 A sagitally acquired STIC volume of the fetal heart and aortic arch at 23w0d. The volume is rendered using the inversion mode and HD*live*, depicting the aortic arch (AoA), descending aorta (DAo), as well as the head and neck vessels (*).

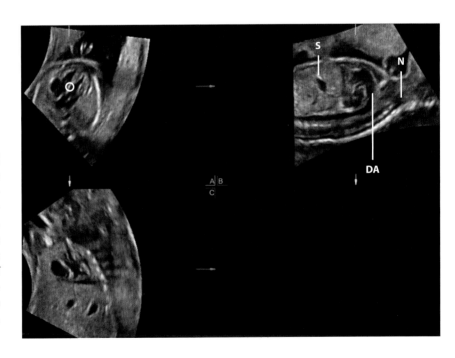

FIGURE 11.7 A 3D volume of the fetal heart at 22w1d is acquired at the level of the four-chamber view with an angle of acquisition of 38 degrees. The volume is subsequently displayed in the multiplanar mode. Note the reference dot (o) at the crux of the heart in plane A. Note that plane B depicts the depth (cephalad and caudad extremes of the acquired volume) and the angle of acquisition, which in this case encompasses the stomach (S) and the neck (N). In addition, plane B depicts the ductal arch (DA).

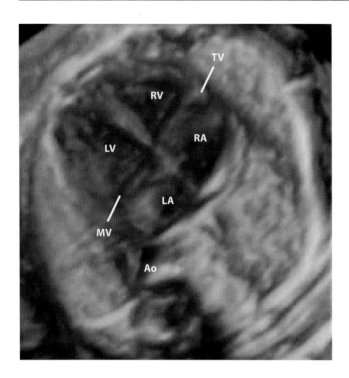

FIGURE 11.8 A 3D volume of the heart of a 29w3d fetus is acquired at the level of the four-chamber view with an angle of acquisition of 53 degrees. The volume is subsequently rendered using surface rendering. Note how clearly the four chambers are seen (RV, right ventricle; LV, left ventricle; RA, right atrium; LA, left atrium), the clear off-setting between the tricuspid (TV) and mitral (MV) valves, and note the left-sided aorta in cross-section (Ao).

A key point for the evaluation of the fetal heart is obtaining the volume with as few extraneous movement artifacts as possible (Table 11.1). Optimizing acquisition, minimizing shadowing from fetal limbs, and standardizing the display are key factors in facilitating navigation through the volume in order to enhance retrieval of the respective anatomic planes out of a stored volume dataset. This was first described by Abuhamad (2004) and is a prerequisite for automation using VCAD (Table 11.2).

Table 11.1 Steps to Obtaining a Standardized Volume of the Fetal Heart

Step 1:	Select the four-chamber view as your reference plane with the ultrasound beam parallel to the ventricular septum
Step 2:	Obtain a 3D sweep with the acquisition box placed just around the heart, with an angle of acquisition of 25 degrees and select a mid to high quality for the volume
Step 3:	Acquire the volume and display it in the multiplanar mode (Figure 11.10)
Step 4:	Rotate the volume in plane A along the Z axis so that the fetal spine is at 6 o'clock and the cardiac apex is in the top left corner
Step 5:	Place the reference dot on the crux of the fetal heart (Figure 11.10)

Table 11.2 Steps to Utilizing VCAD for the Evaluation of the Fetal Heart

Step 1:	Follow steps 1 through 5 to acquire a standardized volume of the fetal heart as described in Table 11.1
Step 2:	Display the volume in the multiplanar mode (Figure 11.10)
Step 3:	Select VCAD as a preset which automatically displays the volume in TUI (Figure 11.11)
Step 4:	Align the four-chamber view with the schematic representation by magnifying the image and rotating it along the Z axis (Figure 11.12)
Step 5:	Align the fetus in plane B with the schematic by rotation along the Z axis (Figure 11.13); this becomes the starting plane (Figure 11.14)
Step 6:	Navigate through the volume, utilizing the predefined cardiac planes 1 through 6 for automatic retrieval of the respective cardiac planes (Figures 11.15–11.20)

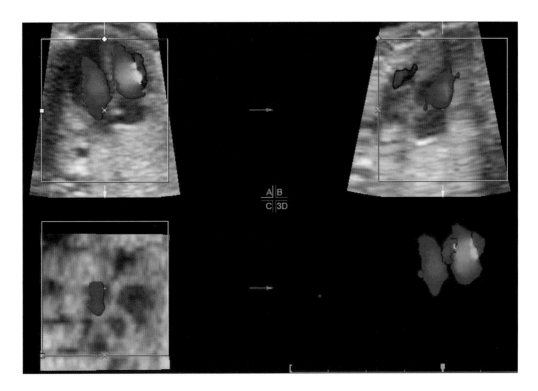

FIGURE 11.9 A STIC volume of the fetal heart at 22w6d is acquired at the level of the four-chamber view with color Doppler. The volume is rendered using minimum mode. The ventricles are clearly depicted.

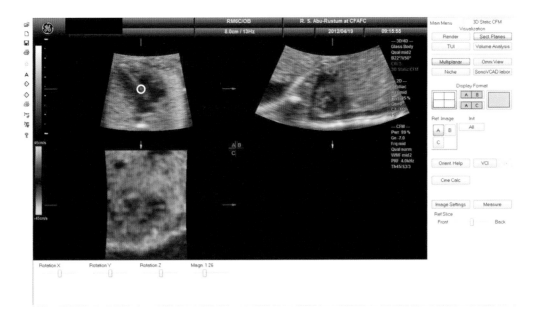

FIGURE 11.10 Figures 11.10–11.20 exemplify the step-by-step approach to utilizing VCAD to generate six cardiac planes out of a 3D stored volume data set of the fetal heart using 4D View software. The first step is to acquire a 3D volume of the fetal heart at the level of the four-chamber view and display it in the three orthogonal planes with the fetal spine at 6 o'clock and the reference dot (O) placed at the crux of the heart as shown in plane A.

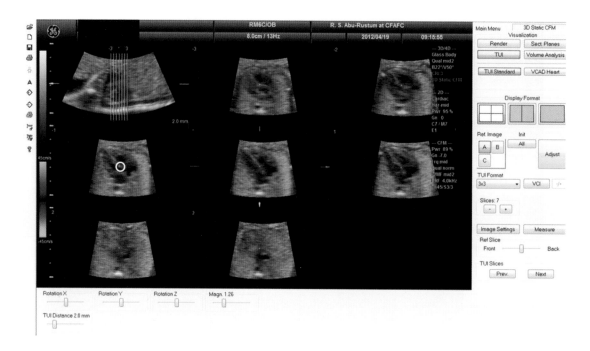

FIGURE 11.11 Subsequently, TUI is selected with seven images at an interslice distance of 2 mm. The reference dot (o) is placed at the crux of the heart.

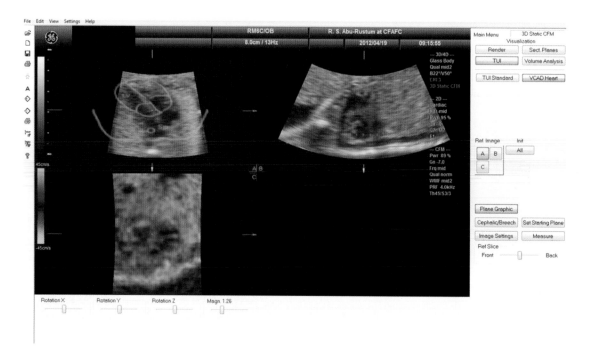

FIGURE 11.12 VCAD is then activated and the diagrams with which to align the images in planes A and B appear. Note the malalignment between the schematic and the sonographic images.

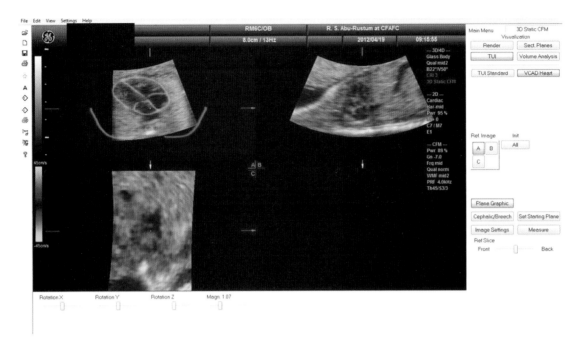

FIGURE 11.13 The image in plane A is then magnified and rotated along the Z axis in order to align it with the schematic, and the image in plane B is rotated in order to align the fetal spine with the dotted schematic line.

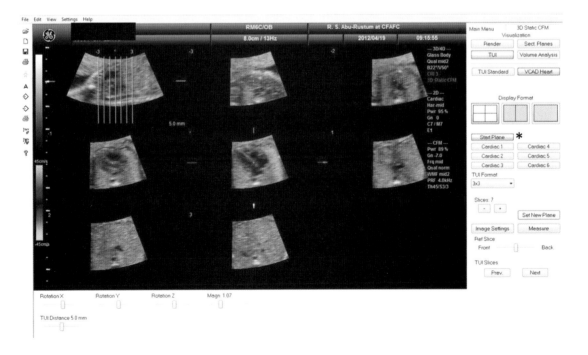

FIGURE 11.14 Once the image has been displayed in the optimal standardized format and aligned with the schematic, the "start plane" button (*) is selected, and now the central image of the four-chamber view becomes the reference plane for navigating within this volume.

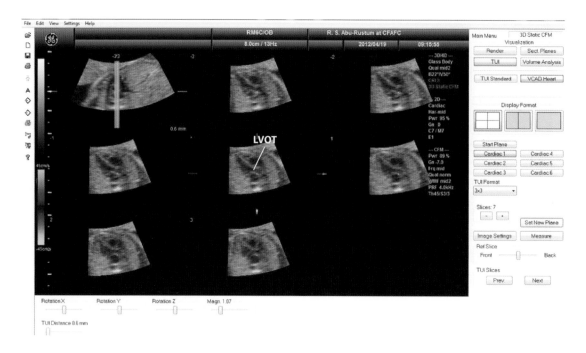

FIGURE 11.15 From the standardized reference plane, the cardiac 1 preset is selected which generates the left ventricular outflow tract (LVOT) in seven planes that are 0.6 mm apart. Utilizing TUI helps correct for the minor variations between fetuses across gestational ages.

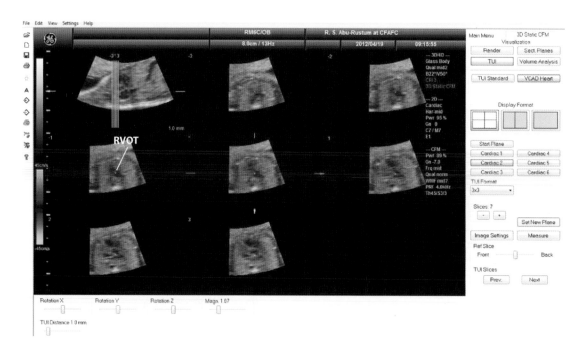

FIGURE 11.16 The cardiac 2 preset is now selected which generates the right ventricular outflow tract (RVOT) in seven planes that are 1 mm apart.

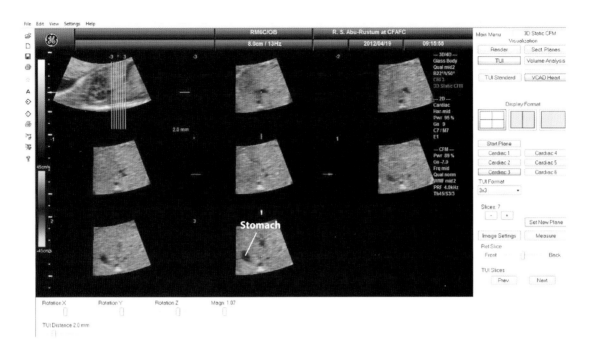

FIGURE 11.17 The cardiac 3 preset is now selected which generates the abdominal circumference plane with a visible fetal stomach. This also helps ascertain fetal situs.

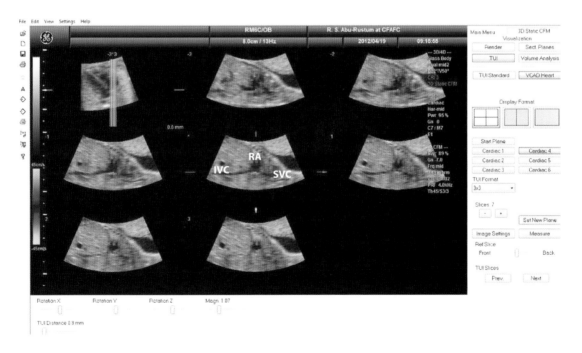

FIGURE 11.18 The cardiac 4 preset is then selected which generates the sagittal views of the right atrial inflow (bicaval view) with the superior and inferior venae cavae (SVC, IVC) inserting into the right atrium (RA).

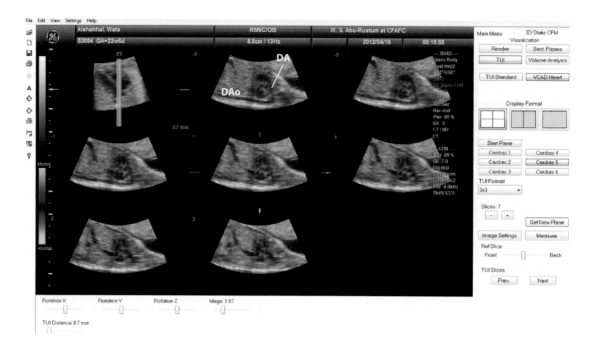

FIGURE 11.19 The cardiac 5 preset is then selected which generates the sagittal views of the ductal arch (DA) and descending aorta (DAo).

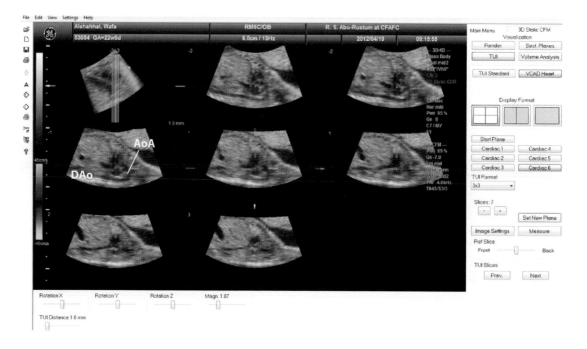

FIGURE 11.20 The cardiac 6 preset is then selected which generates the sagittal views of the aortic arch (AoA) and descending aorta (DAo).

Perhaps the greatest utility for volume sonography in the evaluation of the fetal heart is learning the proper fetal cardiac anatomy and how to generate the necessary cardiac planes out of a standardized volume, to facilitate the evaluation of the fetal heart using 2D ultrasound. It is possible to carry out a near-complete evaluation of the fetal heart from two properly acquired STIC volumes, obtained from an axial and a sagittal sweep, and viewed in cineloop throughout a full cardiac cycle (Figure 11.21 and 11.22). Numerous techniques have been described for studying the fetal heart, including DeVore's spin technique, discussed in Chapter 3 (Table 3.1, Figures 3.17–3.22), study of the fetal valves in Chapter 4 (Table 4.1, Figure 4.3 and 4.4), and Abuhamad's VCAD (Table 11.2, Figures 11.11–11.20), among many others. STIC allows the study of a volume of the beating fetal heart throughout a full cardiac cycle, and combining STIC with TUI, VCI, inversion mode, or any of the Doppler modalities enhances the evaluation (Figure 11.23 and 11.24) and helps reaffirm the location of a ventricular septal defect (Figure 11.25), ventricular (Figure 11.26), and outflow tract abnormalities (Figure 11.27). In addition, STIC has been found to be of value in the off-line analysis of first-trimester normal and abnormal fetal hearts (Chapter 7, Table 7.2, Figures 7.15–7.18) in order to generate the basic views and characterize any underlying pathology. However, as always with volume sonography, the greatest limitation is the quality of the acquired volume and the route of volume acquisitions, whether vaginal or abdominal (Votino et al. 2013). In addition, it is possible to obtain striking surface-rendered images of the fetal heart (Table 11.3).

Table 11.3 **Steps to Acquiring a 3D Surface-Rendered Image of the Four-Chamber View**

Step 1:	Obtain a 3D volume of the fetal heart at the level of the four-chamber view using the cardiac presets and display it in the multiplanar mode (Figure 11.28)
Step 2:	Render the volume using surface rendering with a direction of back-to-front for viewing the region of interest (Figure 11.29)
Step 3:	Change the size of the render box to optimize the final rendered four-chamber view (Figure 11.30)
Step 4:	Select the single-pane display and adjust the threshold and mix (Figure 11.31)
Step 5:	Select HD*live* surface rendering (Figure 11.32)
Step 6:	Adjust the threshold and mix to optimize the texture and appearance of the image (Figure 11.33)
Step 7:	Change the direction of the internal light source in order to reversely illuminate the heart (Figure 11.34)

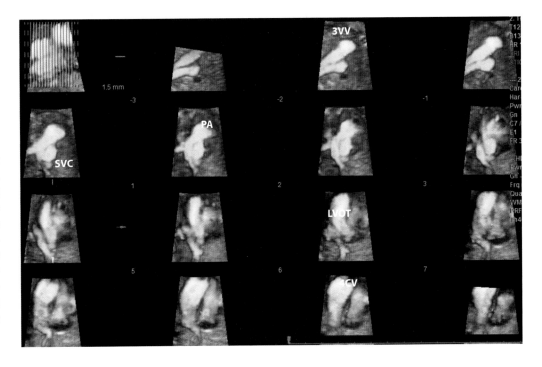

FIGURE 11.21 A STIC volume of a 26w6d heart acquired from the axial plane and displayed using TUI with an interslice distance of 1.5 mm. It is possible to see the four-chamber view (4CV), the left ventricular outflow tract (LVOT), pulmonary artery (PA), three-vessel view (3VV), and superior vena cava (SVC).

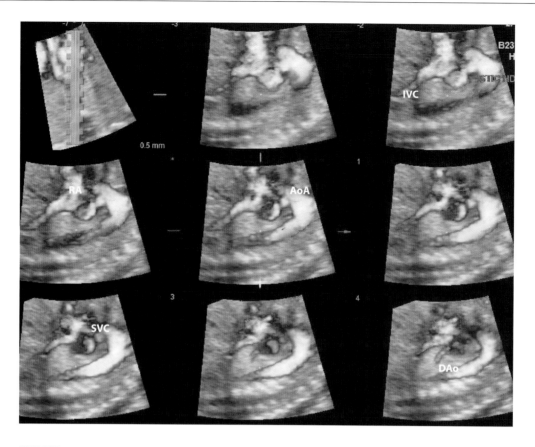

FIGURE 11.22   A sagittally acquired STIC volume of the fetus in Figure 11.21 displayed using TUI with an interslice distance of 0.5 mm. The aortic arch (AoA), descending aorta (DAo), right atrium (RA), and superior and inferior venae cavae (SVC and IVC) can be seen.

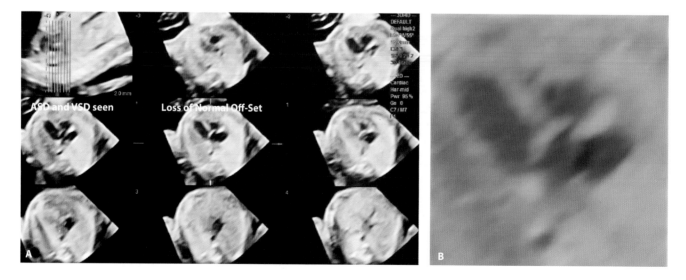

FIGURE 11.23   A 3D volume of a 21w2d fetus with an atrioventricular (AV) septal defect. (A) The volume is displayed using TUI at an interslice thickness of 2 mm and VCI with a slice thickness of 2 mm. The loss of the normal off-set of the AV valves is seen as well as the atrial (ASD) and ventricular (VSD) components of the defect. (B) The volume is rendered using HD*live*, clearly depicting the defect.

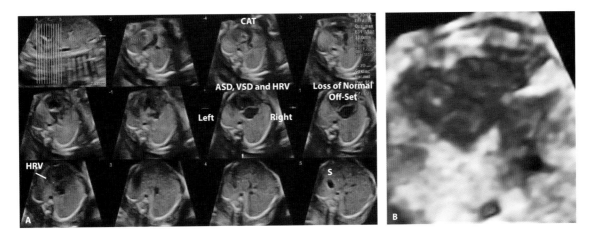

FIGURE 11.24 A STIC volume of a 22w5d fetus with an atrioventricular (AV) septal defect, a hypoplastic right ventricle (HRV), and a common arterial trunk (CAT). (A) The volume is displayed using TUI at an interslice thickness of 2 mm and VCI with a slice thickness of 2 mm. Normal fetal situs is ascertained by visualizing the fetal stomach (S). The loss of the normal off-set of the AV valves is seen as well as the ventricular and atrial components of the defect. (B) The volume is rendered using surface rendering clearly depicting the defect.

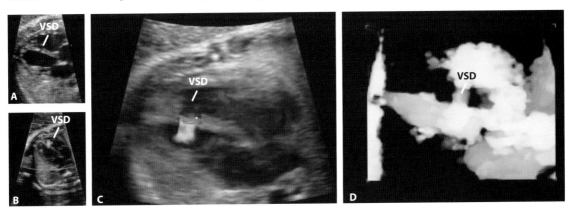

FIGURE 11.25 A series of 2D and 3D images of a second-trimester fetus with an isolated mid-muscular ventricular septal defect (VSD). (A) A 2D image of the four-chamber view depicting the VSD. (B, C) The location of the VSD is ascertained using color Doppler. (D) A 3D volume of the fetal heart is now rendered using the inversion mode, clearly demonstrating the VSD.

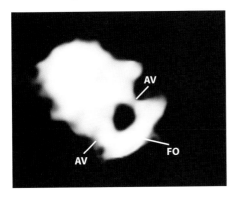

FIGURE 11.26 A 3D volume of a 15w3d fetus with a univentricular heart rendered using the inversion mode during diastole. Note the flow across both atrioventricular valves (AV) as well as across the foramen ovale (FO).

FIGURE 11.27 A 3D sagittal volume of the aortic arch and descending aorta of a 34w0d fetus with ventricular disproportion. The volume is rendered using the inversion mode with HD*live*. This was a case of coarctation of the aorta further clarified utilizing the inversion mode. Note the location of the luminal narrowing (*).

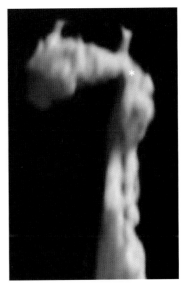

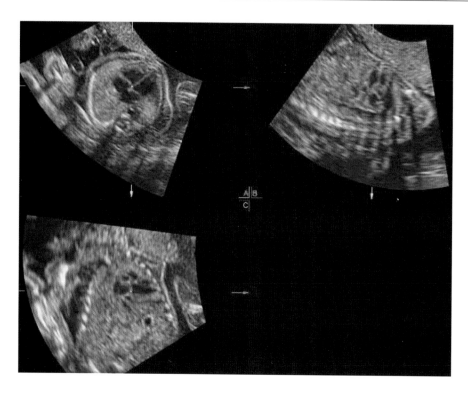

FIGURE 11.28 A 3D volume of the fetal heart at the level of the four-chamber view obtained using the cardiac preset, and displayed in the multiplanar mode.

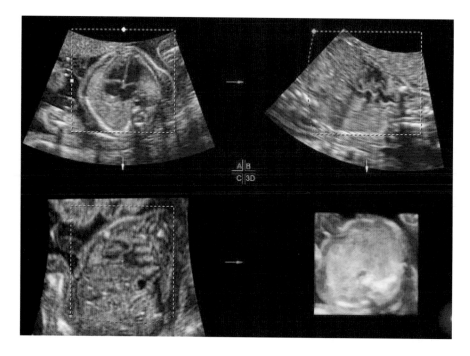

FIGURE 11.29 The volume is rendered using surface rendering with a direction of back-to-front selected in plane B for viewing the region of interest.

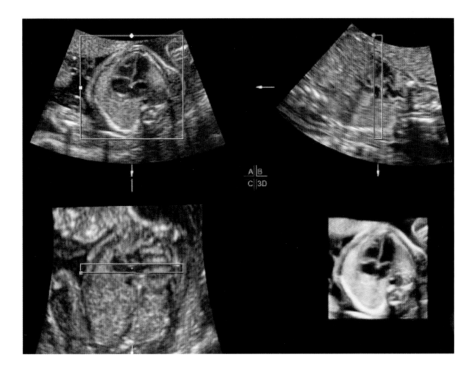

FIGURE 11.30   The size of the render box is adjusted in order to optimize the final rendered image of the four-chamber view.

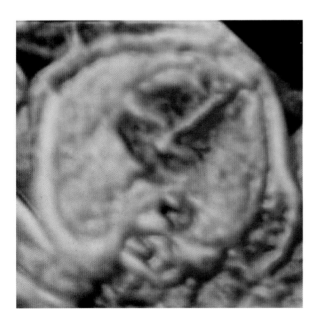

FIGURE 11.31   The single-pane display is selected and the threshold and mix are adjusted in order to optimize the final rendered image.

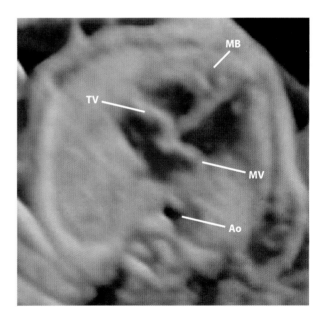

FIGURE 11.32   HD*live* surface rendering is then selected, with which the final rendered image is displayed. Note the left-sided aorta in cross-section (Ao), the normal off-setting of the atrioventricular valves (MV, mitral valve; TV, tricuspid valve), and the thick moderator band (MB) in the right ventricle.

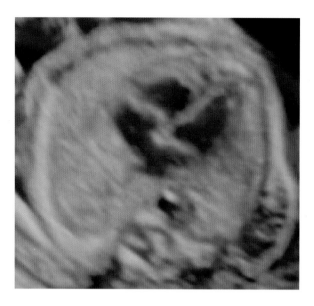

FIGURE 11.33 The threshold and mix are adjusted further in order to change the texture and appearance of the image.

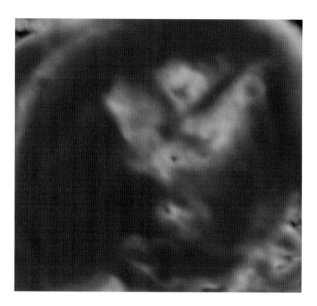

FIGURE 11.34 The direction of the internal light source is changed in order to reversely illuminate the heart.

LIMITATIONS OF VOLUME SONOGRAPHY IN EVALUATION OF THE FETAL HEART

The greatest limitation for the use of volume sonography in the fetal heart is due to the underlying fetal movement which distorts volume imaging, especially in the Y and Z planes. A small angle and the use of STIC can help overcome this limitation to a certain extent. Due to the complexity of the fetal heart, it is easy to get "lost" while navigating through the volume. This is where standardization and the use of the reference dot prove to be of tremendous benefit.

CONCLUSION

Fetal echocardiography remains one of the most difficult areas to perfect as a result of several factors as noted above. With the advent of volume sonography, several modalities are now available to further clarify the area under study and ascertain a diagnosis. This cannot be accomplished without an optimized 2D image from which the volume is obtained. In addition, stored volume datasets of the fetal heart are a great educational tool for the study of normal anatomy and cardiac pathology. With the availability of automation for the second trimester fetal heart on certain sonographic machines, it is now possible to generate all the required key cardiac planes necessary for a complete off-line assessment of the fetal heart out of a standardized stored volume dataset. Ultimately this may translate into better understanding of fetal cardiac anatomy and improved prenatal detection rates.

PRACTICAL PEARLS

- Standardization is key for evaluating the fetal heart
- Any number of modalities may be combined to best evaluate the area in question
- A 15-degree volume angle is sufficient for evaluating the second trimester fetal heart
- Volume sonography provides the best avenue for learning the complicated fetal cardiac anatomy
- During the acquisition of a 3D or STIC volume of the fetal heart, commencing with the four-chamber view, it is possible to view the abdominal circumference plane, four-chamber view, right and left outflow tracts as well as the three-vessel view during the sweep
- It is possible to carry out a complete assessment of the fetal heart from 2 properly acquired STIC volumes: an axial and a sagittal volume

12 Clinical Applicability in the Fetal Chest

INTRODUCTION

The fetal chest is an area that has received much attention with 3D sonography, especially with respect to fetal lung volume measurements. Pulmonary hypoplasia remains a major source of fetal morbidity and mortality. Pulmonary hypoplasia may be the result of several maternal and fetal conditions, oligohydramnios caused by premature rupture of membranes or renal disease, skeletal dysplasias, chylothorax (Figure 12.1), pulmonary masses, and fetal diaphragmatic hernia (Figure 12.2 and 12.3). With the availability of fetal endotracheal occlusion (FETO) for antenatal management of fetal diaphragmatic hernia, lung volume assessments become critical. Fetal lung volumes are calculated pre- and post-FETO for patient selection and for the determination of procedural impact. This has led to several studies investigating the role of volume sonography in accurately quantifying fetal lung volume.

CLINICAL UTILITY

The two main areas of utility of volume sonography in the fetal chest are first, fetal lung development and the establishment of volume normograms, and second, utilizing the various 3D modes to enable more precise diagnoses in fetal lung abnormalities.

AREAS OF UTILITY OF VOLUME SONOGRAPHY IN THE FETAL CHEST

1. Lung development and establishing lung volume normograms
2. Assessing lung abnormalities

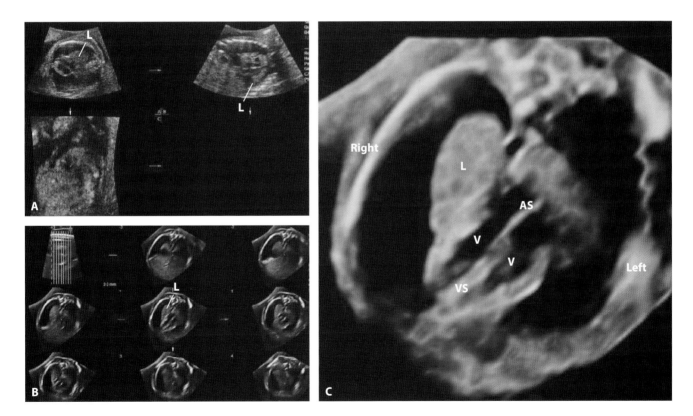

FIGURE 12.1 A 3D volume of the fetal chest of a 20w5d fetus with chylothorax. (A) The volume is displayed in the multiplanar mode using sepia. Note the small fetal lungs (L). (B) The same volume displayed using TUI at an interslice thickness of 3 mm and VCI at a slice thickness of 3 mm, depicting the extent of the chylothorax. (C) A surface-rendered image of the heart and lungs facilitated by the acoustic window created by the fluid filling the chest. V, ventricle; VS, ventricular septum; AS, atrial septum.

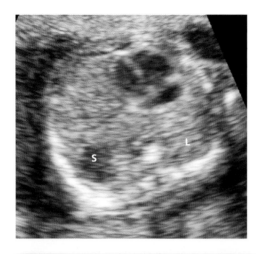

FIGURE 12.2 A 16w6d fetus with a left-sided congenital diaphragmatic hernia. Note the position and axis of the heart now that the abdominal contents have occupied the left side of the chest, with the stomach bubble clearly visible (S). Note the compressed right lung (L).

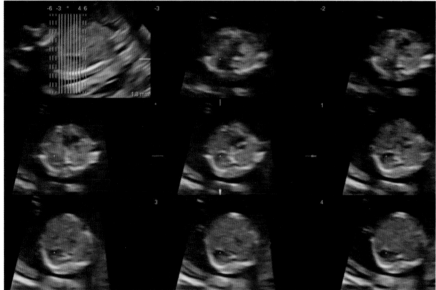

FIGURE 12.3 The same volume from the 16w6d fetus in Figure 12.2 displayed using TUI at an interslice distance of 1.8 mm and a VCI thickness of 1.9 mm. The reference dot is placed within the fetal stomach and locates it in all the planes.

Fetal Lung Volume

There have been numerous studies evaluating the role of volume sonography in determining fetal lung volume, looking at both normal and abnormal lungs, up until gestations of 34 weeks. Beyond 34 weeks, the evaluation becomes very difficult due to a fetal spine-up position, a much larger moving fetal heart, shadowing, and size limitations (Sabogal et al. 2004; Pohls and Rempen 1998). These studies have compared 2D, 3D multiplanar, 3D rotational multiplanar, also known as VOCAL, fetal MRI, and at times have even utilized postmortem lung volumes by water displacement as the gold standard (Pohls and Rempen 1998; Merz 1998; Bahmaie et al. 2000; Osada et al. 2002; Kalache et al. 2003; Sabogal et al. 2004; Ruano et al. 2004a; Moeglin et al. 2005; Ruano et al. 2005a; Peralta et al. 2006a, 2006b; Ruano et al. 2006; Gerards et al. 2006, 2007). Chapter 6 provides a description of fetal lung volume calculation in the case of a normal fetus (Table 6.2; Figures 6.9–6.12). Fetal lung volume measurement in the case of a diaphragmatic hernia is illustrated in Table 12.1 and Figures 12.4–12.8.

Table 12.1 **Steps to Measuring Fetal Lung Volume in Congenital Diaphragmatic Hernia**

Step 1:	Obtain an axial section through the anterior fetal chest at the level of the four-chamber view
Step 2:	Place the acquisition box around the entire chest, with an angle of acquisition of 55 degrees and a mid to high quality for the volume
Step 3:	Acquire the volume and display it in the multiplanar mode (Figure 12.4)
Step 4:	Select VOCAL and use manual trace at a rotational angle of 30 degrees and hit "next" (Figure 12.5)
Step 5:	Point trace the right lung (Figure 12.6) and repeat this step in all six rotational planes
Step 6:	Once the right lung has been traced in all six rotational planes, hit "done" and a 3D reconstruction of the lung appears with the volume calculated (Figure 12.7)
Step 7:	The final rendered volume may be displayed as a mesh and rotated along all three axes (Figure 12.8)

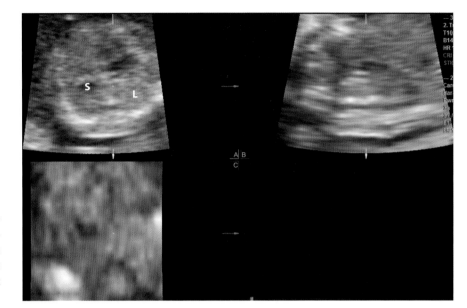

FIGURE 12.4 This is a volume of the same 16w6d fetus with the left-sided congenital diaphragmatic hernia. The volume is displayed in the three orthogonal planes in preparation for calculating the right lung volume.

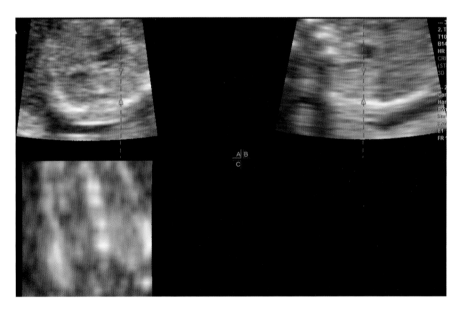

FIGURE 12.5 VOCAL is activated with a rotational axis through the right lung and a rotational angle of 30 degrees. The open arrows are placed along the margins of the right lung.

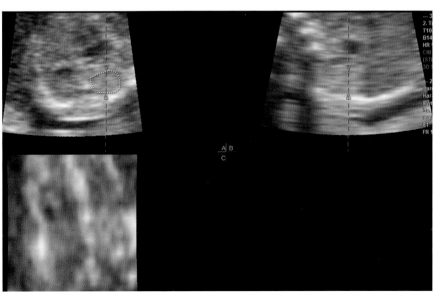

FIGURE 12.6 Manual trace is used to encircle the right lung at a rotational angle of 30 degrees around the vertical axis.

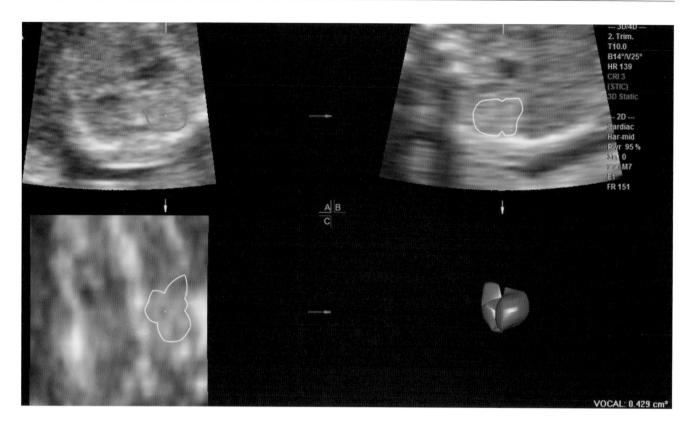

FIGURE 12.7 Once all six measurements are obtained, a 3D schematic of the compressed lung is generated and its volume is calculated: 8.429 cm² in this case.

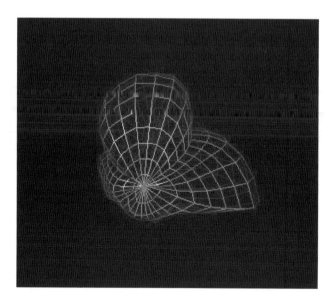

FIGURE 12.8 The final rendered schematic may be displayed in a "mesh" style that can be rotated along any of the three orthogonal axes.

VOLUME SONOGRAPHY IN FETAL LUNG ABNORMALITIES

Another utility of volume sonography is in its role in localizing and evaluating the lungs (Figure 12.9), further characterizing lung lesions and mapping out their extent, involvement of adjacent structures, and their vasculature. A study by Achiron et al. presented an overview of the various modalities in volume sonography and addressed where to use which modality to further enhance the diagnostic accuracy in cases of lung abnormalities (Achiron et al. 2008). Another report by Ruano et al. on a case of a posterior mediastinal lymphangioma concluded that 3D was helpful in determining the precise location of the mass (Ruano et al. 2008). Ruano et al. also investigated the role of 3D power Doppler and found it to be critical in differentiating pulmonary sequestration from congenital cystic adenomatoid malformation of the lung (CCAM) in fetuses with a hyperechogenic lung mass by identifying the feeding vessel. This is helpful in prenatal counseling and postnatal management (Ruano et al. 2005b).

CLINICAL UTILITY OF VOLUME SONOGRAPHY IN LUNG ABNORMALITIES

1. Localizing chest abnormalities
2. Assessing lung abnormalities
3. Differentiating CCAM from pulmonary sequestration

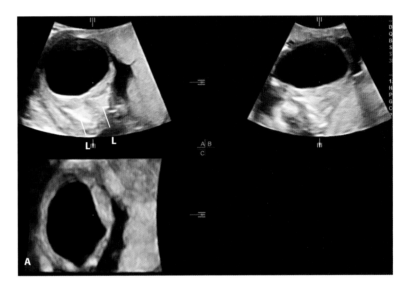

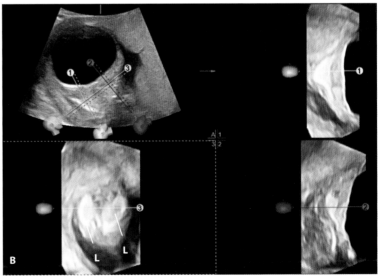

FIGURE 12.9 A 3D coronally displayed volume of a 16w4d fetus with megacystis. (A) The volume is displayed in the multiplanar mode with VCI at a slice thickness of 2 mm. (B) OmniView polyline is activated, with two lines drawn from the apex to the base of each lung and a third line across them, generating three planes in which the fetal lungs are seen.

LIMITATIONS OF VOLUME SONOGRAPHY IN THE EVALUATION OF THE FETAL CHEST

The greatest limitation to using volume sonography in the fetal chest is bone shadowing. This becomes quite challenging beyond 34 weeks of gestation, especially when attempting to calculate fetal lung volumes. It requires skill and practice, and is further limited by suboptimal volumes, especially when there is a structural abnormality.

CONCLUSION

In the assessment of fetal lung volume, 3D ultrasound is most useful, especially in cases of congenital diaphragmatic hernia pre- and post-FETO. It may also be utilized to help in the accurate localization of fetal chest masses and quantifying pleural effusions and chylothorax for monitoring the evolution and progression of pleural effusions and chylothorax. It is of great benefit in learning the anatomy and enabling offline consultation in challenging cases.

PRACTICAL PEARLS

- VOCAL is a most useful modality for quantifying fetal lung volume
- SonoAVC may be used to quantify the amount of chylothorax
- Whenever viewing the heart and lungs from an axially acquired volume, adjust the direction of view of the render box to front-to-back for optimal results
- Avoid acquiring any volumes with fetal extremities covering the fetal chest and use the smallest acquisition box possible
- The 3D techniques are of limited utility beyond 34 weeks due to bone shadowing

13 Clinical Applicability in the Fetal Gastrointestinal Tract

INTRODUCTION

Gastrointestinal abnormalities tend to be identified in the late second and early third trimesters of pregnancy except in cases of abdominal wall defects or hyperechogenic bowel. Similar to the genitourinary tract, the gastrointestinal tract contains several fluid-filled structures. As a consequence, the role of the inversion mode becomes apparent, as does TUI, enabling serial slices spanning the abdominal cavity and pelvis allowing for the characteriztion and accurate identification of the lesion under suspicion.

CLINICAL UTILITY

Most reports on describing the use of volume sonography in evaluating the gastrointestinal tract are limited to case reports in the late second and third trimesters. The main areas of relevance are with respect to quantifying bowel echogenicity, characterizing abdominal wall defects (Figure 13.1 and 13.2), assessing liver volume, and assessing abdominal vasculature, with isolated reports on other gastrointestinal abnormalities (Figures 13.3–13.5).

AREAS IN THE GASTROINTESTINAL TRACT TO BE ASSESSED BY VOLUME SONOGRAPHY

1. Echogenic bowel
2. Abdominal wall defects
3. Liver volume
4. Abdominal vasculature
5. Other areas in the gastrointestinal tract

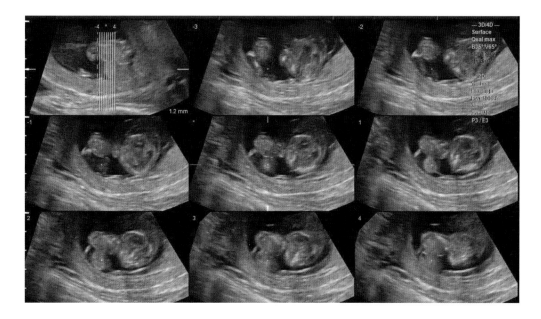

FIGURE 13.1 A sagittal 3D volume of a 11w6d fetus with an omphalocele displayed using TUI at an interslice thickness of 1.2 mm. The reference dot is placed in the fetal omphalocele and localizes it in all the 2D planes.

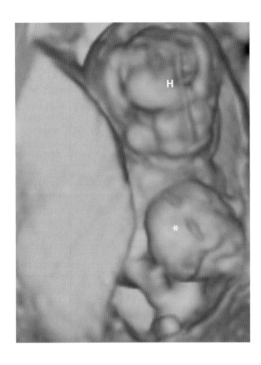

FIGURE 13.2 A 3D volume of a 14w1d fetus with an omphalocele (*) displayed using surface rendering. This 3D image helped clarify the abnormality to the family. H: head.

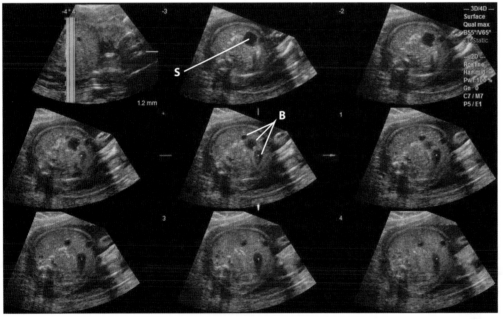

FIGURE 13.3 An axial 3D volume of the fetal abdomen of a 26w1d fetus displayed using TUI at an interslice thickness of 1.2 mm. Note the dilated loops of small bowel, localized by the reference dot. B: bowel; S: stomach.

ECHOGENIC BOWEL

Echogenic bowel is a subjective sonographic finding that is affected by the machine settings, such as employment of tissue harmonics. Its presence may have serious implications since it is a marker for chromosomal aneuploidy, cystic fibrosis, and viral infections. Khandelwal et al. carried out a study on 47 fetuses between 15 and 24 weeks in which an attempt was made to objectively score bowel echogenicity in comparison to bone and the fetal liver, using 3D volumes (Khandelwal et al. 1999). The 3D imaging allowed quantification of the density of bowel, liver, and bone, and it was concluded that comparing bowel to liver echogenicity is of more relevance, whether by 2D or 3D sonography, keeping in mind its wide variability (Figure 13.6). It is this inherent variability that renders the independent use of echogenic bowel unpredictable. As such, when isolated, it is not possible to predict adverse fetal outcome.

CLINICAL UTILITY OF VOLUME SONOGRAPHY IN EVALUATING BOWEL ECHOGENICITY

1. Quantification of bowel density in comparison to liver and bone

---

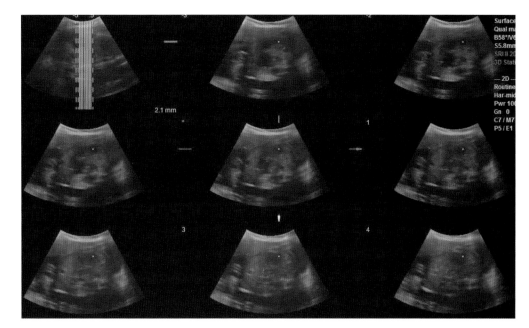

FIGURE 13.4 The same fetus from Figure 13.3 now at 27wld. Again an axial 3D volume of the fetal abdomen is obtained and displayed using TUI at an interslice thickness of 2.1 mm and VCI with a slice thickness of 5.8 mm. The reference dot locates the dilated loop in all the planes.

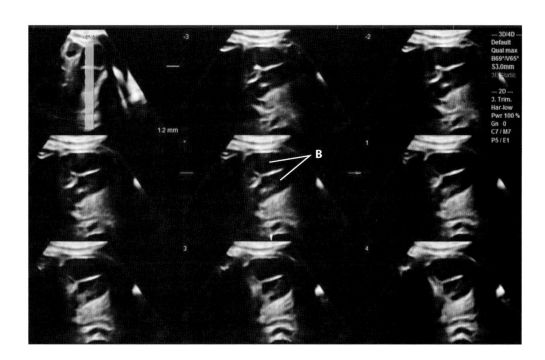

FIGURE 13.5 An axial 3D volume of the same fetus in Figure 13.3 and 13.4, displayed using TUI at an interslice thickness of 1.2 mm with VCI at a thickness of 3 mm. The fetus is now at 37wld. Note the massively dilated small bowel (B).

ABDOMINAL WALL DEFECTS

One of the most investigated areas on the use of volume sonography in the gastrointestinal tract is in cases of abdominal wall defects. In 1996 Matsumi et al. reported on the use of 3D sonography to determine the exact location of abdominal wall defects. (Matsumi et al. 1996). In 2001, Bonilla-Musoles et al. compared the use of 2D to 3D in 12 cases of abdominal wall defects (Bonilla-Musoles et al. 2001). Although 2D allowed better visualization of the herniated contents in the case of an omphalocele, 3D added a great deal of value, especially in the presence of other associated facial anomalies. The final consensus was that the two modalities were complementary, and that the greatest utility for 3D was in

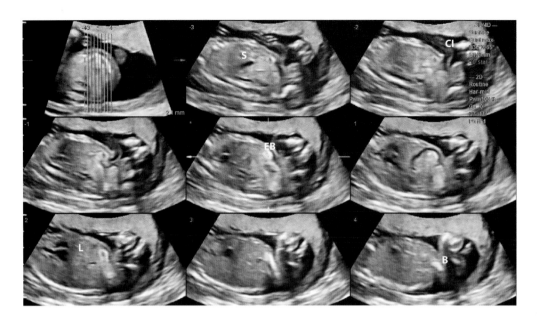

FIGURE 13.6 A sagittal 3D volume of the abdomen and pelvis in a 17w3d fetus. Note the echogenic bowel (EB), which is brighter than the fetal liver (L) and similar in brightness to the fetal bones (B). CI: cord insertion; S: stomach.

the evaluation of fetal gastroschisis prior to 14 weeks of gestation. In early pregnancy, the defect can be infracentimetric, and in the absence of bowel peristalsis the defect may be missed altogether. Anandakumar et al. evaluated volume sonography in a fetus with first-trimester omphalocele and concluded that 3D was able to better clarify and confirm the 2D diagnosis (Anandakumar et al. 2002) (Figure 13.1 and 13.2).

> **CLINICAL UTILITY OF VOLUME SONOGRAPHY IN EVALUATING ABDOMINAL WALL DEFECTS**
>
> 1. Identification of first-trimester abdominal wall defects
> 2. Characterizing the exact location of the lesion
> 3. Identifying other associated anomalies

Liver Volume

Laudy et al. assessed liver volume (Table 13.1; Figures 13.7–13.10) in 34 fetuses at 19–39 weeks and found that liver volume doubled in the latter half of gestation. Liver volume may play a role in identifying fetuses with intrauterine growth restriction (Laudy et al. 1998). Kuno et al. compared 14 appropriately grown fetuses and 10 growth-restricted fetuses to evaluate whether liver volume or length might correlate with intrauterine growth restriction. The study concluded that liver volume, but not liver length, correlated with growth restriction (Kuno et al. 2002).

> **CLINICAL UTILITY OF VOLUME SONOGRAPHY IN EVALUATING LIVER VOLUME**
>
> 1. Calculating liver volume

Table 13.1 **Steps to Measuring Liver Volume**	
Step 1:	Obtain an axial section through the upper abdomen at the level of the abdominal circumference plane
Step 2:	Place the acquisition box around the entire abdomen, with an angle of acquisition of 55 degrees and a mid to high quality for the volume
Step 3:	Acquire the volume and display it in the multiplanar mode (Figure 13.7)
Step 4:	Select VOCAL and use manual trace at a rotational angle of 30 degrees around a rotational *Y* axis that bisects the liver (Figure 13.8) and hit "next"
Step 5:	Trace the liver and repeat this step in all six rotational planes (Figure 13.9)
Step 6:	Once the liver has been traced in all six rotational planes, hit "done" and a 3D reconstruction of the liver appears with the volume calculated (Figure 13.10)

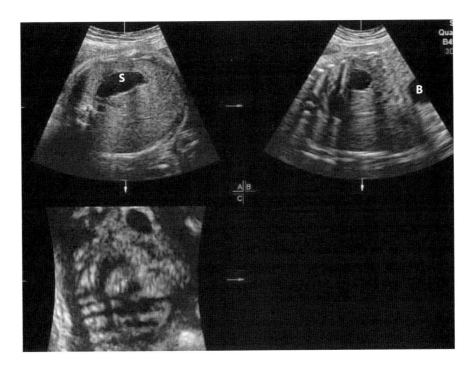

FIGURE 13.7 An axial 3D volume of the abdomen of a 32w1d fetus displayed in the multiplanar mode. B: bladder; S: stomach.

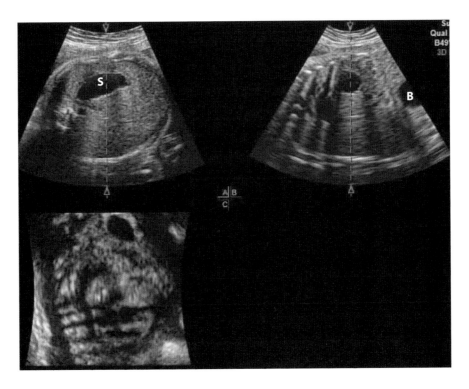

FIGURE 13.8 VOCAL is now selected with a rotational *Y* axis bisecting the fetal abdomen. B: bladder; S: stomach.

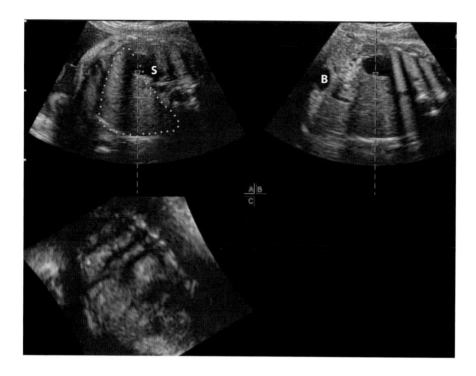

FIGURE 13.9 Manual trace with a rotational angle of 30 degrees is then selected and the fetal liver is traced in six consecutive planes. B: bladder; S: stomach.

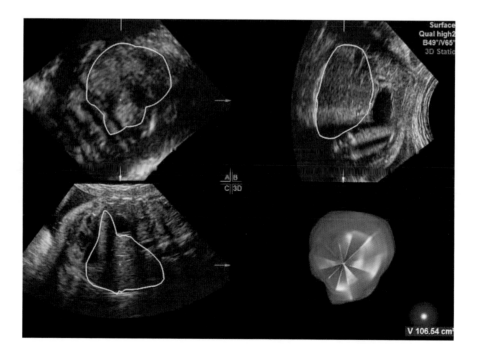

FIGURE 13.10 Once all six measurements are obtained, a 3D schematic of the liver is generated and its volume calculated: 106.54 cm^2 in this case. The final rendered schematic may be rotated along any of the three axes.

ABDOMINAL VASCULATURE

One of the first studies on the use of 3D power Doppler for the study of the fetal abdominal vasculature was by Chaoui et al. where the study was able to differentiate the spleen from the liver and confirm the presence of splenomegaly in a case of cytomegalovirus infection (Chaoui et al. 2002). Paris et al. mapped out the anatomy of the portal sinus using 3D angiography (Paris et al. 2004). Subsequently, Loureiro et al. utilized 3D power Doppler to study the vasculature of a congenital abdominal hemangioma and was able to display the feeding vessel (Loureiro et al. 2008). Sammour et al. diagnosed prenatal volvulus using 3D Doppler, where the 3D counterpart to the 2D "whirlpool sign" was described. This was called the "barber pole" sign (Sammour et al. 2008).

OTHER BENEFITS IN THE GASTROINTESTINAL TRACT

Ramón y Cajal et al. reported on the utility of 3D in differentiating the duodenal and gastric cavities and visualizing the connecting pyloris in a case of duodenal artesia (Ramón y Cajal et al. 2003). Yagel reported on a case of esophageal atresia where 3D facilitated the diagnosis and visualization of the atretic portion of the esophageal pouch (Yagel 2005). Ramon y Cajal et al. reported on visualization of fetal defecation using 4D sonography (Ramón y Cajal et al. 2005). In cases of fetal ascites, the intra-abdominal fluid provides a window through which to obtain nice intra-abdominal images (Figure 13.11 and 13.12).

CLINICAL UTILITY OF VOLUME SONOGRAPHY IN MAPPING OUT ABDOMINAL VASCULATURE

1. Differentiate spleen from liver
2. Map portal sinus angiography
3. Locate the feeding vessel for a hemangioma
4. Identify the "barber pole" sign in prenatal volvulus

OTHER CLINICAL UTILITIES OF VOLUME SONOGRAPHY IN THE GASTROINTESTINAL TRACT

1. Diagnose esophageal atresia
2. Diagnose duodenal atresia
3. Document fetal defecation

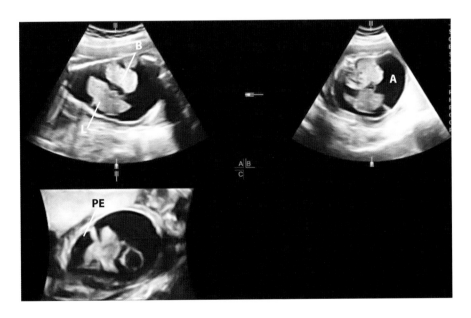

FIGURE 13.11 A 3D volume of 23w2d fetus with ascites displayed using the multiplanar mode with VCI at a thickness of 2 mm. A: ascitis; B: bowel, L: liver; PE: pleural effusion.

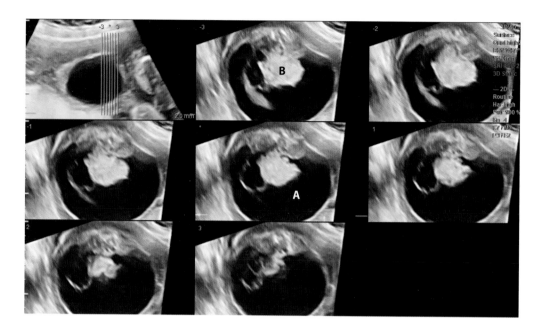

FIGURE 13.12   The same volume from Figure 13.11 now displayed in TUI at an interslice thickness of 2 mm and VCI at a slice thickness of 2 mm, showing the small echogenic bowel and the extent of the ascites. It is possible to use VOCAL in this case to quantify the ascites for follow-up of the progression with advancing gestation. A: ascitis, B: bowel.

LIMITATIONS OF VOLUME SONOGRAPHY IN EVALUATION OF THE GASTROINTESTINAL TRACT

One of the main limitations for the evaluation of the gastrointestinal tract is that most abnormalities are late appearing, first seen in the late second and early third trimesters. At this point in gestation, the 2D scan is more challenging due to fetal flexion and bone shadowing. Since the quality of the 2D image remains the cornerstone for an adequate 3D image, acquisition of an adequate volume with minimal shadowing is the greatest limitation.

CONCLUSION

The gastrointestinal tract remains a challenging area to evaluate, especially in cases of cystic abnormalities. Volume sonography, through the utilization of the inversion mode, TUI, surface rendering, and advanced vascular settings, helps in the clarification of the abnormality present, enhances the diagnostic accuracy, and subsequently may positively impact patient management.

PRACTICAL PEARLS

- When examining the bowel, turn off harmonics, SRI and CRI, especially when evaluating bowel echogenicity
- Volume sonography is most useful in mapping out vasculature and identifying feeding vessels for any masses in the fetal abdomen
- The reference dot proves to be most helpful in the evaluation of cystic abdominal/pelvic lesions while navigating within the volume trying to determine the origin of the lesion

14 Clinical Applicability in the Fetal Genitourinary System

INTRODUCTION

The primary role for volume sonography in the fetal genitourinary system has been gender assignment, renal pelvis volumetry, urine production, and characterizing other genitourinary abnormalities.

CLINICAL UTILITY

As with the gastrointestinal tract, volume sonography plays an important role in the evaluation of the genitourinary tract, especially in the fluid-filled structures, utilizing inversion as well as other 3D modalities.

AREAS IN THE GENITOURINARY TRACT THAT MAY BE EVALUATED BY VOLUME SONOGRAPHY

1. Gender assignment
2. Renal pelvis volumetry
3. Fetal urine production
4. Other areas in the genitourinary system

GENDER ASSIGNMENT

Fetal gender assignment (Figure 14.1 and 14.2) may prove to be difficult especially in the first trimester. The importance of gender assignment is beyond determination of fetal sex; it involves sparing the parents an early CVS in certain X-linked disorders, as well as trying to relieve the stress and serious implications when ambiguous genitalia are suspected. One of the earliest studies on the use of volume sonography for fetal gender assignment was by Hata et al. where 3D sonography was utilized for examining the genitalia in the second and third trimesters (Hata et al. 1998a). A limiting factor in the volumes evaluated in this study was the inability to rotate them, a factor to which the suboptimal results of 3D in comparison to 2D in determining fetal sex may be attributed. Merz et al. reported on a case in which 3D enabled visualization of ambiguous genitalia that were missed on 2D evaluation (Merz et al. 1999). Several studies (Naylor et al. 2001; Cafici and Iglesias 2002; Verwoerd-Dikkeboom et al. 2008; Abu-Rustum and Chaaban 2009) have looked at the role of 3D sonography in cases of ambiguous genitalia. The consensus is that 3D is not diagnostic in cases of ambiguous genitalia but it does help in clarification to the family. Having a multiplanar volume available enables detailed off-line re-evaluation (Abu-Rustum and Chaaban 2009), looking for certain signs such as the tulip sign (Figure 14.3 and 14.4), which is diagnostic in cases of hypospadias. Two recent studies have looked at 3D planes and modes of display to enhance the diagnostic ability of gender assignment. Lev-Toaff et al. reported on using 3D to obtain a true mid-sagittal plane from stored volumes. The true mid-sagittal plane generated was subsequently used to see whether the penis was pointing in a caudal (male) or rostral (female) direction between 10 and 24 weeks (Lev-Toaff et al. 2000). Jouannic et al. reported on utilizing VCI while looking at the pelvis of 38 female fetuses

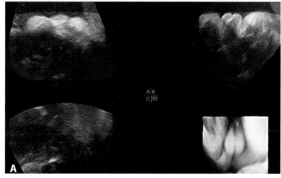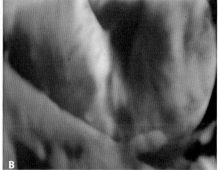

FIGURE 14.1 3D examination of external genitalia. (A) A 3D volume of the external genitalia of a 33w4d female fetus rendered using surface rendering. The labia majora can be depicted with great clarity. (B) A similar volume of a 21w3d fetus displayed using HD*live*.

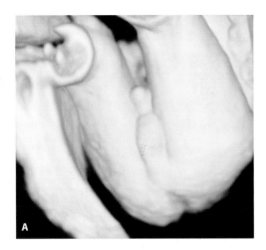
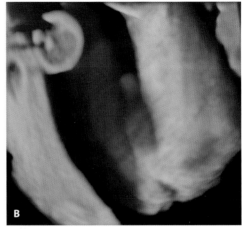

FIGURE 14.2 3D examination of the external genitalia. (A) A 3D volume of the external genitalia of a 27w0d male fetus rendered using surface rendering. The scrotum and penis can be depicted with great clarity. (B) The volume is now displayed using HD*live*.

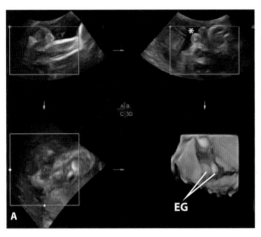
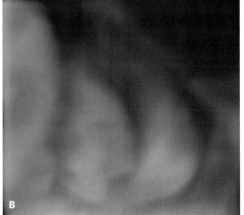

FIGURE 14.3 3D examination of ambiguous external fetal genitalia (EG). (A) A 3D volume of the external genitalia of a 34w5d fetus displayed using surface rendering with HD*live*. The 2D image in plane A depicts the "tulip" sign described in hypospadius. The 3D surface-rendered image was highly suggestive of swollen labia in a female fetus. (B) A close-up of the external genitalia. This fetus was a live born male with hypospadias.

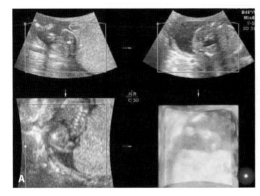
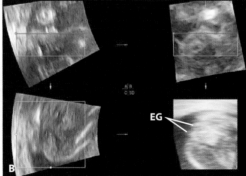

FIGURE 14.4 A 22w3d fetus with multiple anomalies. (A) A 3D volume of ambiguous external genitalia (EG) is acquired and displayed using surface rendering. (B) The Volume is manipulated by adjusting the size of the render box and rotating along the three axes. Surface rendering is used, depicting seemingly female external genitalia. However, postmortem this was a male fetus with hypospadias and a bifid scrotum.

at 20–22 and 32–34 weeks in an attempt to further enhance the endometrial visualization. The VCI mode clarified the distinction between the uterus and rectum (Jouannic et al. 2005).

UTILITY OF VOLUME SONOGRAPHY IN THE EVALUATION OF FETAL GENDER

1. Clarifying ambiguous genitalia
2. Utilizing the mid-sagittal plane for first-trimester sex determination
3. Utilizing VCI for the clarification of the endometrial stripe

---

RENAL PELVIS

Hydronephrosis (Figure 14.5) is a marker for chromosomal aberrations and exists in a continuum of gradations. It may be benign or it may signal underlying renal disease, from uretropelvic junction obstruction in its varying degrees, to reflux. Measuring the anteroposterior diameter of the renal pelvis has been the gold standard, but with the advent of volume sonography, the volume of the renal pelvis can now be measured. Duin et al. succeeded in measuring the volume of the fetal renal pelvis in 15 fetuses and found it feasible and reproducible, but in need of comparison to the standard anteroposterior measurement to determine its clinical utility (Duin et al. 2008). In addition, the inversion mode may be of great use in mapping out the entire pelvis and calyceal system in cases of hydronephrosis (Table 14.1; Figures 14.6–14.8) and in creating a true cast of the calyceal system.

UTILITY OF VOLUME SONOGRAPHY IN THE EVALUATION OF THE RENAL PELVIS

1. Calculating the volume of the renal pelvis
2. Mapping the architecture using inversion mode

FIGURE 14.5 A 3D volume of the left kidney of a 34w1d fetus with hydronephrosis. Using the inversion mode and adjusting the threshold, it is possible to generate a "cast" of the renal pelvis (P) and calyceal system (*). It would be possible to utilize VOCAL as well for volume calculation.

FETAL URINE PRODUCTION

The amniotic fluid index may be measured in several ways, and the importance of quantifying the amniotic fluid lies in its ability to indicate adequate fetal vascularization, in the absence of fetal hypoxia, reflected by good urine production. However, the amniotic fluid is not made up entirely of urine, and there have been various attempts at quantifying the amount of fetal urine production more accurately, an area in which volume sonography has played a role. Lee et al. examined 154 fetuses, between 24 and 40 weeks, and employed VOCAL in order to measure the fetal bladder volume two to three times within a 5–10 minute period. The mean fetal bladder volume was plotted against the gestational age. This may be an alternative method for quantifying the amniotic fluid index, and it may aid in signaling fetal hypoxia (Lee et al. 2007). Similarly, Yamamato et al. looked at fetal urine production using VOCAL in 106 twin-to-twin-transfusion syndrome cases, pre- and post-laser, to determine how it correlated with umbilical venous volume flow. The conclusion was that urine production is a useful tool in assessing the severity of twin-to-twin-transfusion syndrome (Yamamato et al. 2007).

UTILITY OF VOLUME SONOGRAPHY IN THE EVALUATION OF FETAL URINE PRODUCTION

1. Quantifying urine production

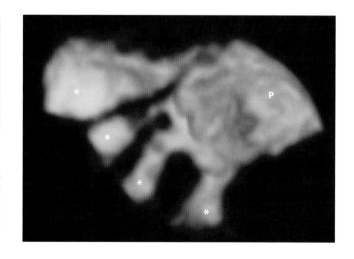

Table 14.1 Steps to Mapping the Fetal Renal Calyceal System

Step 1:	Obtain a volume of the fetal kidneys starting from an axial plane with an angle of acquisition of at least 30 degrees
Step 2:	Optimize the volume in planes A and B by rotating along the 3 axes to optimize the views of the renal pelvis (Figure 14.6)
Step 3:	Select the two-pane view and render the volume using surface rendering
Step 4:	Adjust the threshold to create the optimal inverted image (Figure 14.7)
Step 5:	The volume may also be rendered using HD*live* inversion (Figure 14.8)

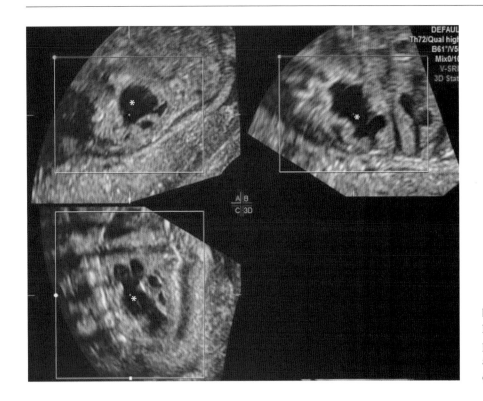

FIGURE 14.6 A 3D volume of the left kidney of a 31w4d fetus with hydronephrosis (*). The volume is acquired with an angle of acquisition of 55 degrees and displayed in the three orthogonal planes.

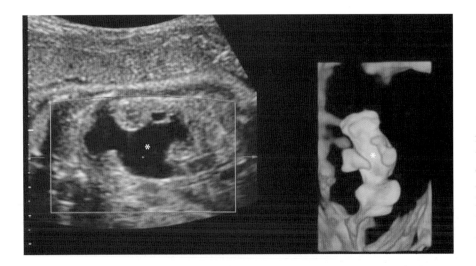

FIGURE 14.7 This is the same volume from Figure 14.6. Now the two-pane view is selected and rotation is carried out along the three axes, with the region of interest concentrated around the kidney to be examined. The volume is then rendered using the inversion mode in surface rendering, as seen in panel B. Renal pelvis (*).

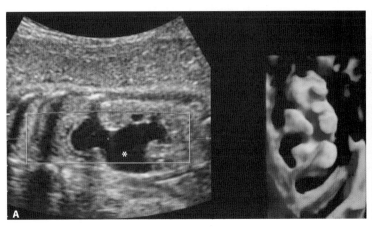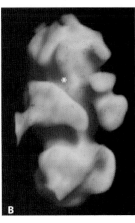

FIGURE 14.8 The same volume as in Figure 14.6 and 14.7. (A) The volume is displayed using HD*live* inversion mode. (B) The volume is viewed in the single-pane view, and using MagiCut, all excess material obscuring the kidney is removed for an optimal final "cast" of the calyceal system under evaluation. Renal pelvis (*).

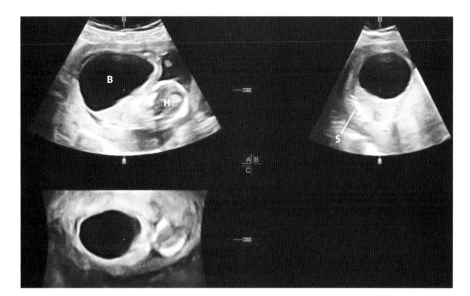

FIGURE 14.9 A 3D volume of a 15w4d fetus with megacystis displayed using the multiplanar mode with VCI at a slice thickness of 2 mm. B: bladder C: chest; H: head; S: spine.

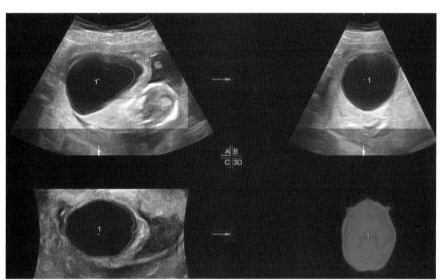

FIGURE 14.10 This is the same volume as in Figure 14.9, now being evaluated using SonoAVC with automatic generation of the volume of the fetal bladder of 47.51 cm².

OTHER USES IN THE GENITOURINARY TRACT

Schild et al. reported on the use of 3D in a case of fetal mesoblastic nephroma that was initially diagnosed as a Wilms' tumor. The 3D imaging allowed volume calculation and a reliable estimation of the size of the mass as well as characterization of the borders of the mass (Schild et al. 2000). Dulay et al. reported on the use of 3D in a case of vesicorectal fistula in cloacal dysgenesis. The 3D imaging was key in identifying the bladder with the umbilical arteries, as demonstrated by color Doppler, and in finding the connection between the bladder and bowel by scrolling through the volume (Dulay et al. 2006). Hsu et al. found 3D power Doppler helpful in localizing an aberrant renal artery arising from the iliac artery and feeding the kidney's inferior pole. Aberrant renal arteries may be a normal variant and may arise from the aorta. In this case, combining 2D and 3D power angiography allowed the diagnosis of a horseshoe kidney (Hsu et al. 2007). Most recently, Ruano et

al. used 4D sonography in a case of fetal lower urinary tract obstruction as a guide to percutaneous cystoscopy, and this was the first fetal cystoscopy under 4D guidance (Ruano et al. 2009). Volume sonography may also help in the evaluation of the fetus with megacystis (Figures 14.9–14.11).

**OTHER USES OF VOLUME
SONOGRAPHY IN THE EVALUATION
OF THE GENITOURINARY TRACT**

1. In the evaluation of tumors
2. In the evaluation of a fistula
3. In the evaluation of an ectopic kidney
4. In guidance during fetal cystoscopy
5. In the evaluation of megacystis

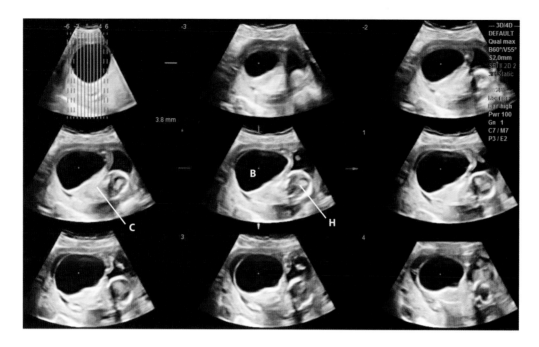

FIGURE 14.11   This is the same volume from Figure 14.9. The volume is now displayed using TUI with an interslice thickness of 3.8 mm and a VCI thickness of 2 mm, with the reference dot in the fetal bladder. B: bladder; C: chest; H: head.

LIMITATIONS OF VOLUME SONOGRAPHY IN THE EVALUATION OF THE GENITOURINARY SYSTEM

The major limitation with volume sonography in the genitourinary system is false diagnoses, especially in cases of ambiguous genitalia. Therefore the examiner needs to carry out a meticulous evaluation, relying on internal as well as external 2D findings, prior to announcing the fetal gender to the family based solely on a 3D surface-rendered image.

CONCLUSION

Volume sonography has several key roles in the evaluation of the fetal genitourinary system. Surface rendering aids in visualizing the external genitalia; however, navigating through a volume, looking for other signs such as the tulip sign and the distance between the bladder and rectum (Glanc et al. 2007), provides more conclusive information. In addition, volume sonography, utilizing inversion mode as well as VOCAL, aids in evaluating the fetal calyceal system in cases of hydronephrosis, and may help in quantifying urine production.

PRACTICAL PEARLS

- In order to visualize the kidneys, OmniView may be utilized commencing with an axial plane in order to generate coronal or sagittal views of the kidneys
- Inversion mode is most useful in mapping out the fetal calyceal system
- VCI is helpful in the evaluation of fetal hydronephrosis
- Minimum and inversion modes are helpful in the evaluation of the kidneys and bladder

15 3D Applications in Obstetrics

INTRODUCTION

In addition to what has already been discussed, there are constantly emerging studies pertaining to the various applications of volume sonography in obstetrics. The focus of this chapter is therefore on other clinical applications of 3D ultrasound in obstetrics.

OTHER APPLICATIONS OF VOLUME SONOGRAPHY IN OBSTETRICS

1. Placenta and cord
2. Fetal weight estimation
3. Fetal behavior
4. Review of topographic anatomy
5. Intrapartum role

CLINICAL UTILITY

The utility of volume sonography in various aspects of obstetrical sonography is now discussed, keeping in mind that new roles are constantly undergoing assessment and evaluation.

PLACENTA AND CORD

Volume sonography can be an added benefit in several areas, including evaluation of placental masses, placental localization for suspected placenta previa (Figure 15.1), and whenever there may be retained products of conception (Figure 15.2). Volume sonography is also helpful in ascertaining the number of cord loops (Figure 15.3) or true knots in the cord (Figure 15.4) whenever these abnormalities are suspected.

ROLE OF VOLUME SONOGRAPHY IN THE EVALUATION OF THE PLACENTA AND CORD

1. Placental masses
2. Placental localization
3. Retained products of conception
4. Nuchal cord
5. True knot in the cord

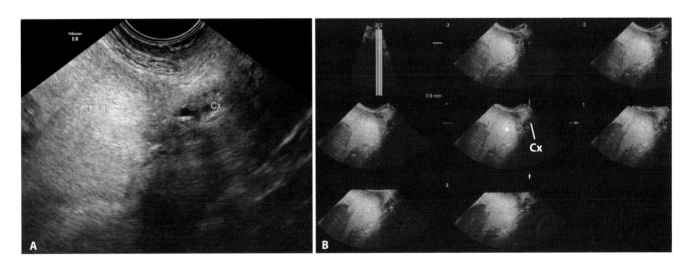

FIGURE 15.1 A 12w6d intrauterine pregnancy with a suspected placenta previa. (A) Transvaginal evaluation reveals a central previa completely covering the internal cervical os (Cx). (B) A 3D transvaginal volume of the uterus is displayed utilizing TUI at an interslice distance of 0.8 mm, further ascertaining the central location of the placenta previa (*).

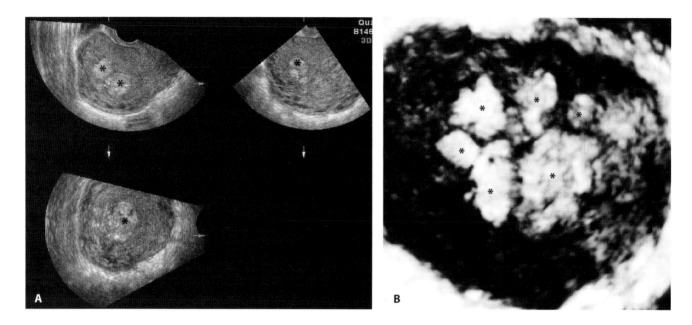

FIGURE 15.2 A 3D transvaginally acquired volume of a postpartum uterus with retained products of conception (*). (A) The volume is displayed in the multiplanar mode, clearly depicting retained placental products. (B) Surface rendering is utilized to display the volume. The threshold and mix are adjusted to highlight the retained placental products, which are often challenging to depict with conventional 2D sonography.

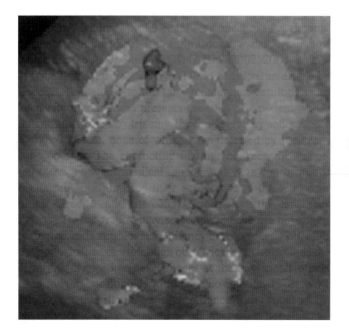

FIGURE 15.3 A 3D volume of a suspected entangled cord at 35w6d utilizing color Doppler. Glass-body mode is used, highlighting the vascular structures and clarifying the entangled cord.

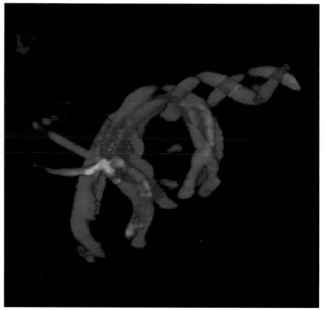

FIGURE 15.4 A 3D volume of a 27w3d intrauterine pregnancy with a true knot in the cord. The volume is displayed in the 3D CFM mode, which highlights the vascular structure, illustrating the knot in the cord.

ESTIMATION OF FETAL WEIGHT

A novel application for volume sonography, which has been studied by Lee et al. (2001b, 2009), is the use of fetal arm and leg volumes to assist in the accurate estimation of fetal weight. This application has been developed into a software program currently available on certain machines. A stepwise approach on how to calculate fetal weight from the fetal thigh is described in Table 15.1. In a recent study by Pagani et al., its use in fetal weight estimation in mothers with gestational diabetes mellitus was found to be of comparable sensitivity but of superior specificity in fetal weight estimation at 34w0d–36w6d when compared to the conventional Hadlock formula for predicting fetal macrosomia (Pagani et al. 2014).

Table 15.1 **Steps to Utilizing Fractional Limb Volume**

Step 1:	Obtain a good 2D image of the fetal thigh
Step 2:	Acquire a 3D volume utilizing the surface-rendering machine preset and place the reference dot centrally along the femur (Figure 15.5)
Step 3:	Select the FLV option (Figure 15.6)
Step 4:	Trace the cross-sections of the fetal thigh sequentially as prompted by the program (Figure 15.7)
Step 5:	Once all tracings are complete, a thigh volume (TVol) will be obtained from which the fetal weight is automatically generated (Figure 15.8)

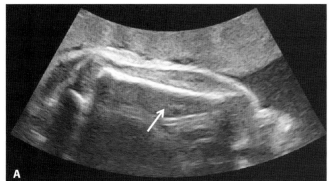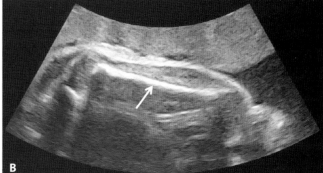

FIGURE 15.5 A 3D volume of a fetal thigh at 31w3d displayed in a single pane (plane of acquisition plane A) of the multiplanar mode. (A) The original volume with the arrow pointing to the reference dot. (B) The reference dot (arrow) has now been moved to a central position along the midpoint of the fetal femur.

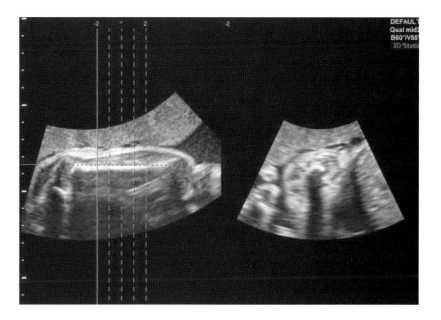

FIGURE 15.6 The fractional limb volume software has now been activated generating five axial slices of the fetal thigh in order to calculate the limb volume.

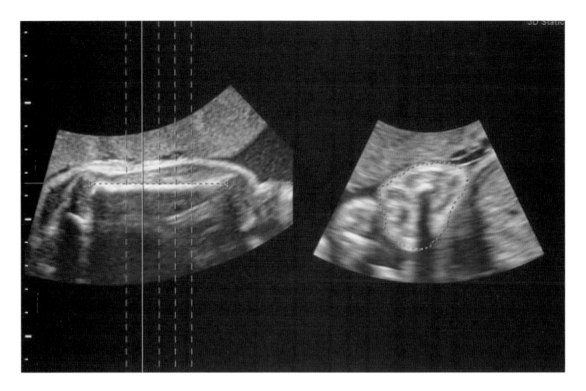

FIGURE 15.7 Using the area trace, the circumference of the fetal thigh is encircled sequentially in each of the five generated volumes.

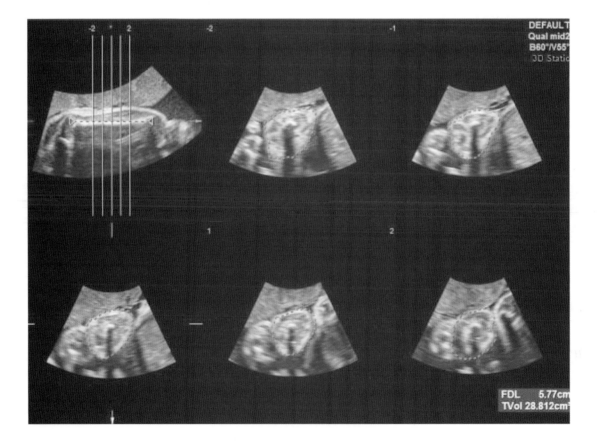

FIGURE 15.8 Once all five tracings are complete, the system displays the tracings in a single view with an automatically generated fractional limb volume from which the fetal weight is generated.

Fetal Behavior

The role of volume sonography for the evaluation of the fetal surface, specifically for the visualization of facial grimaces and detailed limb movements, has been evaluated by Kurjak et al. to assess fetal neurobehavior (Kurjak et al. 2010), attempting to identify fetuses with abnormal in utero neurologic function. The authors employed the Kurjak Antenatal Neurodevelopmental Test in which 4D ultrasound was employed to score fetuses based on the presence of various facial grimaces and movements (Figures 15.9–15.13).

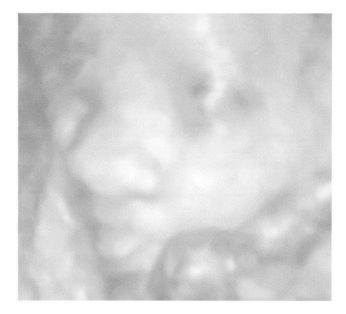

FIGURE 15.9 A 3D surface-rendered image of a 29w0d fetal face with the fetal tongue sticking out.

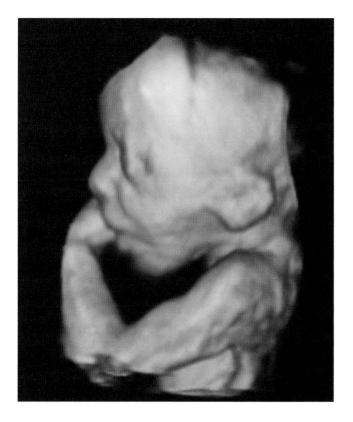

FIGURE 15.10 A 3D surface-rendered image of a 21w5d fetus sucking his thumb.

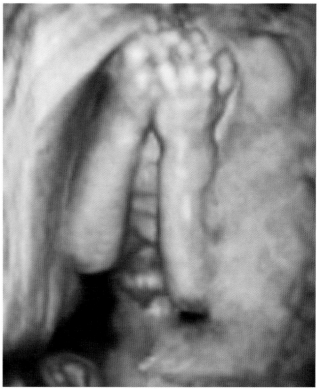

FIGURE 15.11 A 3D surface-rendered image of a 23w5d fetus hiding its face behind both hands.

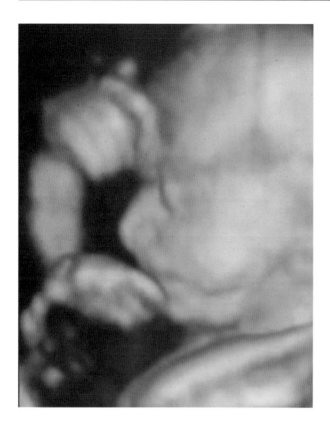

FIGURE 15.12 A 3D surface-rendered image of a 24w0d fetus scratching its head.

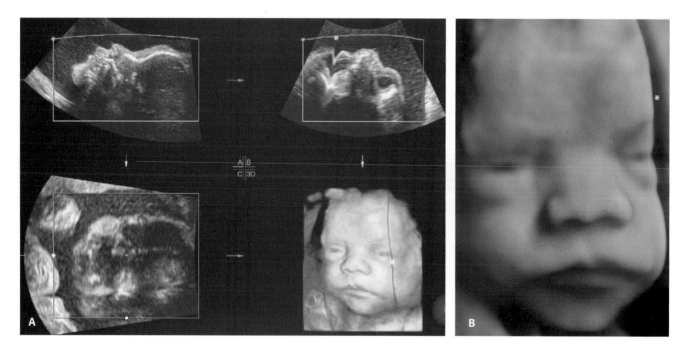

FIGURE 15.13 A 3D surface-rendered volume of a 30w1d fetus with open eyes. Note artifact (*) generated by fetal movement. (A) The volume is displayed in the multiplanar mode with surface rendering. (B) The volume is rendered with HD*live*.

REVIEW OF TOPOGRAPHIC ANATOMY

The role of volume sonography in the review of topographic anatomy has been assessed, and it was found to be useful in the evaluation of first trimester losses. For instance, in a case of a missed abortion, 3D ultrasound identified the presence of conjoined twins, otherwise missed by conventional 2D ultrasound, at a challenging early point in gestation where the patient had presented with fetal demise (Abu-Rustum and Adra 2007) (Figure 15.14). In addition, a study by Bromley et al. found it to be of benefit in the evaluation of fetuses presenting with first trimester demise as it helped clarify various external structural abnormalities that were otherwise missed by 2D ultrasound (Bromley et al. 2010).

INTRAPARTUM ROLE

The role of volume sonography in assessing the position of the fetal head during labor has been studied by several experts, at the forefront of which is Pilu's group, leading to the development of the SonoVCAD*labor* software to monitor fetal head progression in the birth canal during labor (Ghi et al. 2010). It has recently been shown that there is a good correlation between 2D and 3D sonography in the evaluation of the head-to-symphysis distance (Youssef 2013).

LIMITATIONS OF VOLUME SONOGRAPHY IN OBSTETRICS

The major limitation to utilizing these various applications of 3D ultrasound in obstetrics remains the steep learning curve, in addition to added cost of some of the software mentioned.

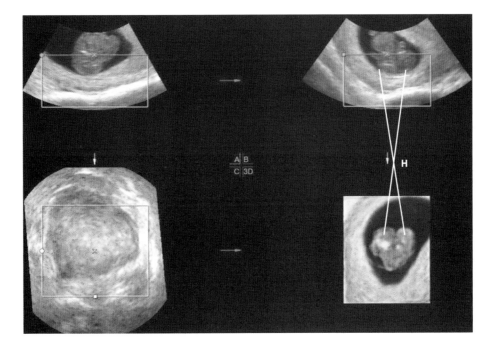

FIGURE 15.14   A transvaginally acquired 3D surface-rendered volume of a missed abortion at 10w3d in which a round mass was seen next to the fetal head. 3D was of tremendous value in this case of first trimester fetal demise, as it demonstrated a case of conjoined twins as seen in the final-rendered image. H: fetal head.

CONCLUSION

The role of volume sonography has encompassed every aspect of obstetrics including fetal organ system assessment, the study of in utero fetal behavior, placental assessment, fetal weight estimation, topographic evaluation in the case of fetal demise, and monitoring fetal head progression during labor. The future will undoubtedly bring more applications integrating the benefits of volume sonography together with automation. The optimized acquired 2D image remains the basis for a good 3D volume. Volume sonography will never replace conventional 2D ultrasound, but it plays an important complementary role.

PRACTICAL PEARLS

- When uncertain about placental location, obtain a volume and scroll through it or utilize TUI to ascertain the distance of the placental edge from the internal os
- When in doubt concerning a knot in the cord, a volume with color Doppler may help clarify whether or not it is present
- Even in the case of a first trimester fetal demise, obtaining a 3D volume may prove to be of utility in providing an explanation as to the cause of the demise

16 3D Applications in Gynecology

INTRODUCTION

Traditionally, we have been limited in how we evaluate the pelvic organs by the available transabdominal and transvaginal routes and the angles from which we can visualize them. Using traditional 2D approaches, there are several questions that can be posed and the two most relevant are:

1. Are the angles used to acquire the 2D images optimal?
2. How feasible is it to obtain a true coronal view of the uterus?

The answers to the above questions were elegantly discussed by Benacerraf in her lecture "Viewing the Dark Side of the Moon" (oral communication International Society of Ultrasound in Obstetrics and Gynecology World Congress 2004), in which she addressed these issues and how with volume sonography we may now gain access to these organs through never-before-used image planes that more accurately depict pelvic anatomy. The benefits of volume sonography in gynecology extend far beyond the uterus; they encompass evaluation of the adnexa in polycystic ovaries, evaluation of follicles in assisted reproduction, characterization of benign ovarian cysts (Figure 16.1), differentiation of hydrosalpinx from an ovarian cyst, evaluation of tuboovarian abscesses, paraovarian cysts, and gynecologic tumors. Additional information can be obtained with volume sonography when performing saline infusion sonohysterography (Figure 16.2) and hysterosalpingo-contrast-sonography (Benacerraf et al. 2005; Bocca et al. 2012; Bocca and Abuhamad 2013; Sakhel et al. 2013). Because motion and motion artifacts are not a concern, gynecological volumes can be acquired with the highest quality, generating images with superb resolution, which are further enhanced when utilizing high-frequency transvaginal probes.

With volume sonography, we may also standardize the acquisition of a uterine volume and subsequently manipulate the volume using Abuhamad's Z technique (Abuhamad et al. 2006) (Table 16.1) to obtain the perfect coronal view. This has gained momentum as an effective, cost-containing, invaluable modality in the diagnosis of müllerian anomalies (Bocca et al. 2012; Bocca and Abuhamad 2013; Sakhel et al. 2013).

CLINICAL UTILITY

There are many benefits to utilizing volume sonography in the field of gynecology.

CLINICAL UTILITY OF VOLUME SONOGRAPHY IN GYNECOLOGY

1. Characterizing uterine pathology
2. Visualizing the mid-coronal plane of the uterus
3. Counting follicles in assisted reproduction
4. Differentiating ovarian from tubal pathology
5. Characterizing gynecologic tumors
6. Enhancing the visualization in sonohysterography
7. Other utilities

UTERINE PATHOLOGY

Volume sonography can provide a great deal of detail when evaluating the endometrium and the uterus for the presence of uterine fibroids (Figure 16.3). It facilitates determining the extent of their intramural extension and enables better typing and management.

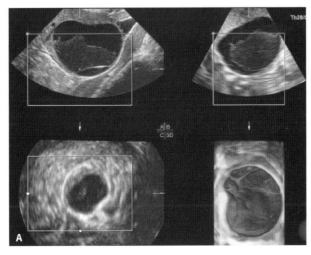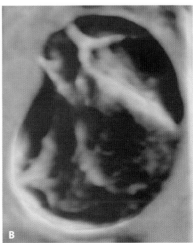

FIGURE 16.1 A transvaginal 3D volume of a hemorrhagic ovarian cyst is obtained. (A) The volume is displayed in the multiplanar mode with surface rendering. (B) The final rendered volume using HD*live* is displayed where the fibrous mesh within the cyst is clearly depicted.

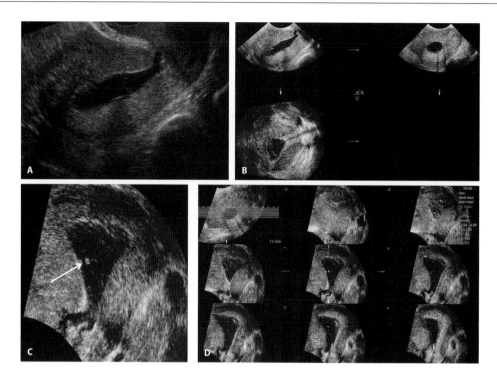

FIGURE 16.2 A transvaginal sonohysterography with saline infusion. (A) 2D sagittal image of the fluid-filled endometrial cavity is obtained. (B) Volume of the uterus is now acquired and is displayed in the three orthogonal planes. (C) Rotation along the *X*, *Y*, and *Z* axes has been carried out, and the single pane has been chosen. Note the catheter tip (arrow). (D) The volume is now displayed using TUI at an interslice distance of 1.5 mm, allowing for a more comprehensive evaluation of the normal endometrial cavity.

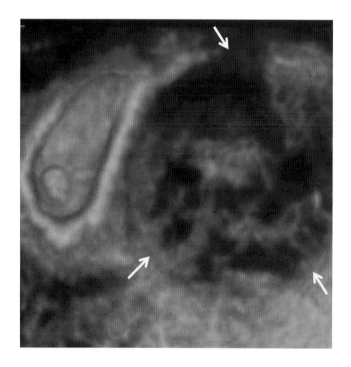

FIGURE 16.3 A transabdominal 3D volume of a 10w1d intrauterine pregnancy displayed using surface rendering, with a leiomyoma (arrows) seen abutting the gestational sac.

MID-CORONAL PLANE OF THE UTERUS

The mid-coronal plane of the uterus is of utmost importance, and it is inaccessible using traditional 2D sonography. With volume sonography, the acquisition of this plane becomes a possibility and facilitates evaluation of several key constituents in gynecology, primarily in the evaluation of müllerian anomalies. There is ample evidence today in support of the reliable, cost-effective, safe, and well-tolerated use of 3D ultrasound in comparison to hysterosalpingography in the evaluation of müllerian abnormalities. Utilizing Abuhamad's *Z* technique (Table 16.1; Figures 16.4–16.9) (Abuhamad et al. 2006), Bocca et al. were able to demonstrate that 3D ultrasound is effective and accurate when compared to hysterosalpingography, at less cost and morbidity to the patient, for the evaluation of müllerian anomalies (Bocca et al. 2012).

MAIN ADVANTAGES OF THE MID-CORONAL PLANE OF THE UTERUS

1. Evaluating the serosal fundus
2. Evaluating the endometrial fundus
3. Evaluating the lower segment

Table 16.1 **Steps to Utilizing the Z Technique to Obtain the Mid-Coronal View of the Uterus**

Step 1:	Obtain a 3D volume of the uterus starting from the sagittal plane (Figure 16.4)
Step 2:	Display the volume in the multiplanar mode (Figure 16.5)
Step 3:	Place the reference dot in the center of the endometrial stripe in plane A (Figure 16.6)
Step 4:	Align the sagittal plane to depict the endometrial stripe as horizontally as possible in plane A by rotating along the Z axis (Figure 16.7)
Step 5:	Select plane B and rotate along the Z axis in order to align the endometrial stripe horizontally (Figure 16.8)
Step 6:	The mid-coronal plane will be automatically displayed in plane C and may be optimized by rotation along the Z axis (Figure 16.9)

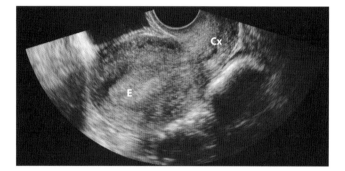

FIGURE 16.4 The first step for employing the Z technique is to obtain a transvaginal 3D volume of the uterus, commencing with the sagittal plane. In this volume, VCI was used at a slice thickness of 1 mm. Cx: cervix; E: endometrium.

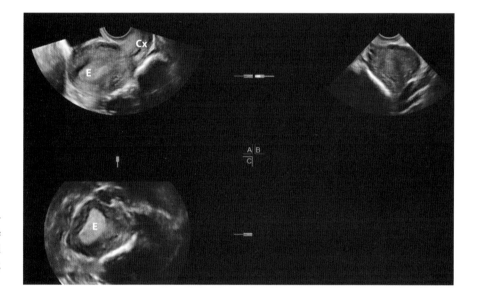

FIGURE 16.5 The volume is then displayed in the multiplanar mode. Note the position of the reference dot, which shall be key in the subsequent steps. Cx: cervix; E: endometrium.

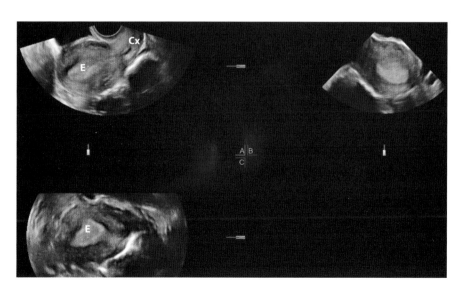

FIGURE 16.6 The reference dot is then placed centrally along the endometrial stripe in plane A. Cx: cervix; E: endometrium.

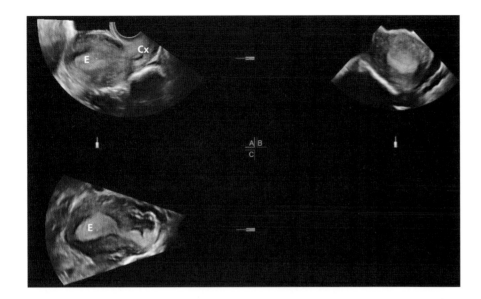

FIGURE 16.7 Rotation along the Z axis is then carried out in plane A to align the endometrial stripe in as horizontal a lie as possible. Cx: cervix; E: endometrium.

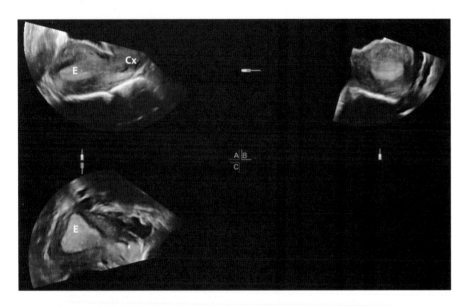

FIGURE 16.8 Plane B is then selected and Z rotation is carried out to align the endometrial stripe horizontally. This automatically generates the coronal view of the endometrial cavity in plane C. Cx: cervix; E: endometrium.

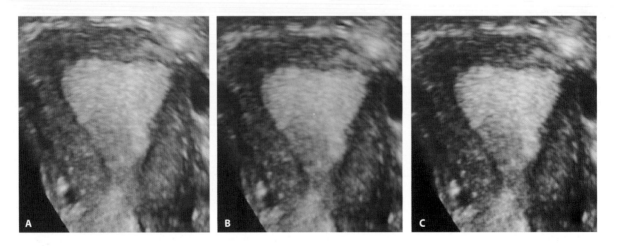

FIGURE 16.9 Coronal view of the uterus. (A,B,C) Plane C is selected and rotation along the Z axis is then carried out to orient the endometrial cavity in its normal anatomical position. The image threshold, transparency, and color are adjusted to optimize the depiction of the coronal view of the uterine cavity.

Assisted Reproduction

One of the greatest roles for volume sonography has been in assisted reproduction, particularly in tracking ovarian follicles. This has been facilitated through the use of SonoAVC. Obtaining a 3D volume of an ovary and activating SonoAVC makes it possible to automatically color-code, count, and calculate the volume of all the follicles within an ovary, thus facilitating optimal management of patients undergoing ovarian stimulation and properly timing oocyte retrieval. The steps for using inversion on a cystic ovary and SonoAVC to calculate follicular number and volume were covered in Chapters 4 and 6 (Tables 4.2 and 6.3; Figure 4.12 and Figures 6.13–6.15).

Adnexal/Gynecological Pathology

Volume sonography provides clarification of the characteristics of all gynecological tumors to help differentiate benign from malignant tumors. By utilizing the various rendering techniques, it is possible to visualize hair within mature teratomas (Figure 16.10), excrescences (Figure 16.11), and obtain 3D renderings to study complex vascularity. In addition, evaluating tubal pathology and differentiating tubal (Figure 16.12) from ovarian pathology (Figure 16.13) is greatly facilitated.

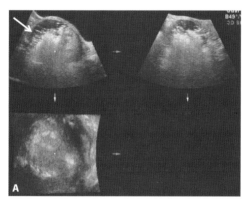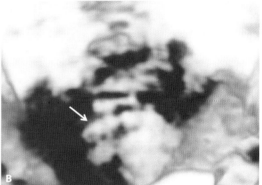

FIGURE 16.10 A transabdominal 3D volume of a mature teratoma. (A) The volume is displayed in the multiplanar mode. Note the hair filaments in plane A (arrow). (B) The volume is rendered depicting the mixed nature of the constituents of the cyst, with visible hair filaments now having a thicker appearance (arrow).

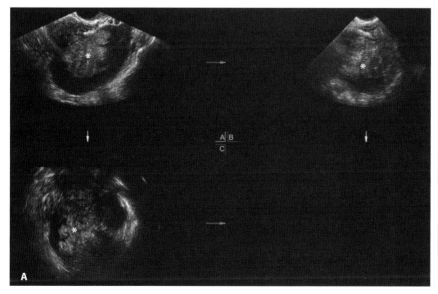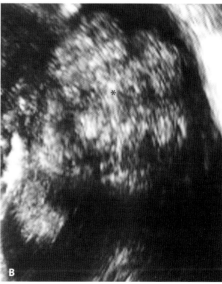

FIGURE 16.11 A transvaginal 3D volume of an ovarian tumor is obtained. (A) The volume is displayed in the multiplanar mode. (B) The volume is rendered using surface rendering, depicting the solid nature of the mass with excrescences (*).

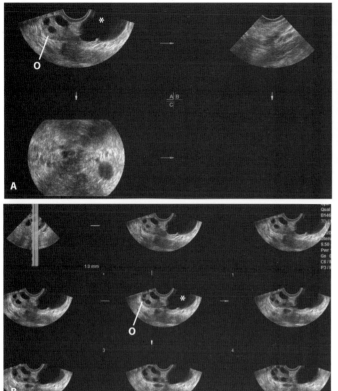

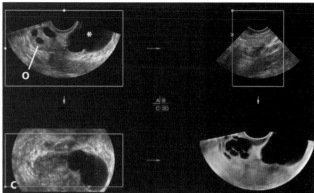

FIGURE 16.12 A transvaginal 3D volume of the right adnexa. (A) The volume is displayed in the multiplanar mode. (B) The volume is displayed using TUI at an interslice distance of 1 mm, clearly demonstrating that the cystic tubular structure (*) is separate from the ovary (O). (C) The volume is rendered using the minimum mode. All the above 3D modalities, together with rotation along the three orthogonal planes, depict a tubular structure, separate from the ovary, and thus help confirm the diagnosis of a hydrosalpinx.

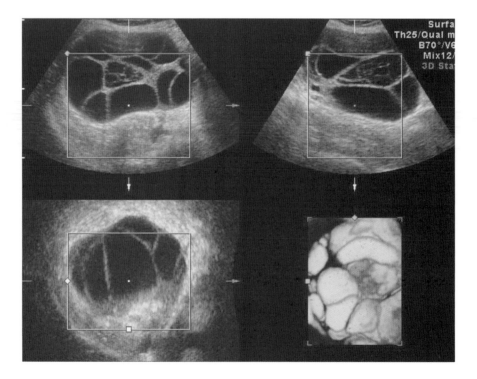

FIGURE 16.13 A transvaginal 3D volume of the adnexa displayed using inversion mode, depicting multiple follicles in a patient with hyperstimulation syndrome.

SONOHYSTEROGRAPHY

The availability of volume sonography coupled with sonohysterography has had a positive impact on the evaluation of the endometrium, and on localizing and characterizing endometrial polyps (Figure 16.14). The proper utilization of these two modalities may save the patient having to undergo other more costly procedures such as a hysterosalpingography.

OTHER USES

Localizing intrauterine devices has always been a challenge with 2D sonography and other imaging modalities are frequently needed to determine whether an intrauterine device has slipped or is properly placed. This is especially applicable in cases of unexplained pelvic pain. However, with the availability of volume sonography and proper use of the Z technique, it is possible to properly ascertain the intrauterine device's location using ultrasound as a single imaging modality (Figures 16.15–16.17) (Sakhel et al. 2013).

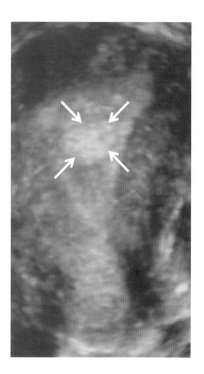

FIGURE 16.14 A transvaginal 3D volume of the coronal view of the endometrial cavity displayed using VCI at a slice thickness of 4 mm, depicting a hyperechogenic central area, an endometrial polyp (arrows).

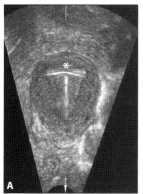
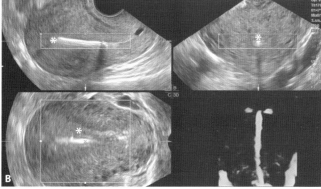
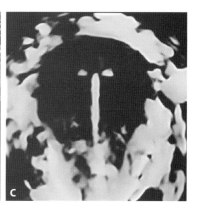

FIGURE 16.15 A transvaginal 3D volume of the endometrial cavity from two patients displayed in the coronal view, illustrating a perfectly placed intrauterine device (IUD) (*). (A) Final surface-rendered coronal plane of patient 1. (B) Volume of patient 2 displayed in the three orthogonal planes and rendered with the minimum mode. (C) Final rendered image of patient 2 using minimum mode where the color settings have been adjusted, clearly displaying the proper placement and the shape of the Cu-T 380A IUD.

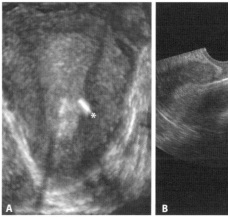
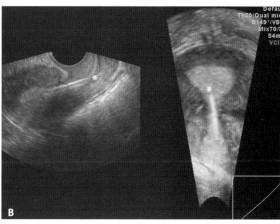

FIGURE 16.16 Transvaginal coronal view of the endometrial cavity for localization of an intrauterine device (IUD) (*). (A) A slipped intrauterine device shown using the Z technique. (B) Another slipped intrauterine device displayed utilizing VCI at a thickness of 4 mm.

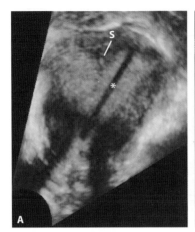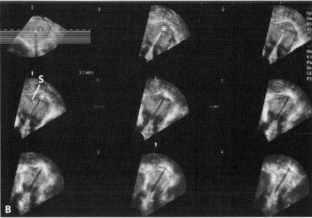

FIGURE 16.17   Transvaginal coronal view of the endometrial cavity for the localization of an intrauterine device (IUD) (*). (A) Utilizing the Z technique demonstrates a uterine septum with the IUD to the left of the septum. (B) Employing TUI at an interslice thickness of 3.1 mm and VCI at a slice thickness of 3.4 mm generates a clear depiction of the endometrial cavity, the septum (S), and the location of the IUD.

LIMITATIONS OF VOLUME SONOGRAPHY IN GYNECOLOGY

As described by Nelson et al., artifacts are as apparent in volume sonography as in 2D ultrasound, and the presence of the third dimension may compound the artifact (Nelson et al. 2000). This is why the basic gold standard to a good 3D image remains an underlying good 2D image. Nonetheless, it must be kept in mind that there are limiting factors to the utility of volume sonography in gynecology as summarized below.

> **LIMITING FACTORS TO VOLUME SONOGRAPHY IN GYNECOLOGY**
>
> 1. Inability to determine uterine orientation
> 2. Poor rotation may show pathology in cases of a normal uterus
> 3. An off-center tilt may also show pathology in cases of a normal uterus
> 4. Often times, the cervix and uterus may not be in the same plane

CONCLUSION

The role of 3D ultrasound in gynecology has not been utilized to its maximal potential, and with proper training it is an invaluable diagnostic tool to the practicing gynecologist and anyone involved in gynecological imaging. Over the past few years, several reports have provided ample evidence in support of its utility as a first-line modality for the diagnosis of uterine anomalies. Global governing bodies, at the forefront of which is the American Institute of Ultrasound Medicine, are advocating its use by raising awareness and providing proper guidance and training to caregivers.

PRACTICAL PEARLS

- The key to a good 3D image is a good 2D image
- Since motion artifacts are not a concern, use maximal quality and a wide angle when acquiring a volume of the uterus and adnexa
- In gynecology, penetration mode, CRI (compound resolution imaging), and harmonics may be helpful
- In order to surface-render the endometrium, the reference box should be minimized along the desired area of the endometrium and then surface-rendered in any of several modes
- For the best endometrial assessment, scan during the secretory phase, day 14–28 (Benacerraf oral communication 2007)
- For performing a sonohysterography, scan prior to ovulation, day 5–12 (Benacerraf oral communication 2007)
- For evaluating the postmenopausal endometrium, scan any time (Benacerraf oral communication 2007)
- For inversion of a fluid-filled area, such as in sonohysterography or in the case of a hydrosalpinx, optimize contrast resolution and use the transparency mode for best image quality

17 Coding and Entertainment Ultrasound

INTRODUCTION

Volume sonography requires time and dedication to develop the necessary skill and to employ the various 3D modalities available. However, 2D ultrasound remains the "gold standard," where in experienced hands its use is sufficient to arrive at the most complicated diagnoses. Because of this, billing and third-party coverage for 3D ultrasound continue to face major limitations. Although the practitioner may bill for a 3D sonographic examination, reimbursement, unless for specific indications, remains minimal.

CODING

Performing a 3D examination requires costly sonographic equipment in addition to a steep learning curve for the practitioner. It also requires time allocation during the examination and additional time is required for off-line analysis after completion of the examination. With limited reimbursement, this is a major challenge hindering the widespread use of 3D ultrasound in obstetrics and gynecology (Ob/Gyn).

INDICATIONS FOR POTENTIAL REIMBURSEMENT IN 3D SONOGRAPHY

1. Skeletal abnormalities
2. Facial anomalies
3. Uterine anomalies

Coding in Ob/Gyn Sonography

There are various codes that may be used in Ob/Gyn sonography. Tables 17.1 and 17.2 list the major codes with their requirements (GE Healthcare 2011; United Healthcare 2013; AIUM 2014) for the United States.

Table 17.1 Various CPT Codes in Gynecological Sonography

CPT 76856	Complete pelvic, nonobstetric, real-time examination with image documentation
CPT 76857	Limited or follow-up pelvic, nonobstetric, real-time examination with image documentation (for instance, for follicular monitoring)

Coding in 3D Sonography

Although CPT codes for 3D ultrasound have been introduced, reimbursement remains minimal and there is a consensus among global organizations such as the American Institute of Ultrasound in Medicine (AIUM) (http://www.aium.org), the Society for Maternal-Fetal Medicine (SMFM) (http://www.smfm.org), and the American Congress of Obstetricians and Gynecologists (ACOG) (http://www.acog.org) in North America that unless medically indicated, there should be no billing for a 3D scan. The physician may still choose to obtain 3D images for the patient at no additional cost. However, for certain indications where there is sufficient evidence of the added benefits of 3D ultrasound, it may be possible to bill using the 3D ultrasound-specific codes (Table 17.3) (APS Medical Billing 2013).

There are many resources available pertaining to coding in obstetrics and gynecology, and recent comprehensive online

Table 17.2 Various CPT Codes in Obstetrical Sonography

CPT 76801	Transabdominal first trimester (<14w0d) fetal and maternal evaluation of a single or first gestation. Use CPT +76802 for each additional gestation
CPT 76805	Transabdominal fetal and maternal evaluation (> 14w0d) of a single or first gestation. Use CPT +76810 for each additional gestation
CPT 76811	An indication-based examination not for routine use in all pregnancies. To be used once per pregnancy. Use CPT +76812 for each additional gestation
CPT 76813	Transabdominal or transvaginal evaluation with nuchal translucency measurement for a single or first gestation. Use CPT +76814 for each additional gestation
CPR 76815	Limited evaluation of the fetal heartbeat, placental location, fetal position, and amniotic fluid index on 1 or more fetuses
CPT 76816	If 76811 did not allow a full evaluation, a focused reassessment may be planned and code 76816 may be used for the follow-up examination
CPT 76817	Transvaginal evaluation with image documentation
CPT 76820	Fetal and umbilical artery Doppler velocimetry
CPT 76821	Fetal middle cerebral artery velocimetry
CPT 76825	Echocardiography (2D) with or without M-mode recording
CPT 76826	Follow up or repeat to CPT 76825
CPT 76827	Complete Doppler echocardiography
CPT 76828	Follow up to CPT 76827

resources are available through the AIUM and other organizations (GE Healthcare 2011; United Healthcare 2013; APS Medical Billing 2013; AIUM 2014).

Table 17.3	**Various CPT Codes in 3D Sonography**
CPT 76376	3D rendering with post-processing interpretation; however, not requiring post-processing on a separate workstation
CPT 76377	3D rendering with post-processing interpretation; however, requiring post-processing on a separate workstation

"ENTERTAINMENT ULTRASOUND"

At the conclusion of this guide on volume sonography, having discussed all the basic aspects of the various techniques and where and how to utilize them, there must be a brief closing discussion on "entertainment ultrasound." This nonmedical use of ultrasound, also known as "keepsake" imaging, has tainted the image of volume sonography. As the practitioner commences on incorporating volume sonography into daily clinical practice, it is critical to maintain focus on the key constituents of a thorough obstetrical evaluation without losing sight of what is important, by misusing resources for the sake of "pretty" images and perhaps falsely reassuring patients about the health and well-being of their fetuses.

Several press releases and position statements have been issued by leading professional organizations cautioning against the nonmedical use of ultrasound, at the forefront of which are the AIUM and ACOG (AIUM 2002, 2004, 2005a, 2005b, 2005c, 2012; ACOG 2004). In addition, an article by Greene et al. attests to the false reassurance resulting from keepsake imaging and presents the case of a patient whose fetus was affected by trisomy 18 with seven key sonographic markers present, none of which were detected by the keepsake scanner. The conflicting findings between the "entertainment" and the "medical" sonograms were confusing for the family and hindered their acceptance of the fetal condition (Greene and Platt 2005). Nonetheless, the consensus is that 3D sonography may serve to enhance the physician-patient relationship. Therefore it may be a consideration, after the performance of a thorough obstetrical scan, to provide the family with nice keepsake images at the physician's office, time and fetal position permitting, at no additional cost to the family, but this should be in accordance with proper medical practice, while enhancing physician–patient bonding and ensuring patient satisfaction.

CONCLUSION

Despite the role of 3D ultrasound in clarifying various fetal structural defects and its role in the evaluation of the uterine cavity, reimbursement for an examination that requires costlier machines, more operator skill, and more time allocation remains the greatest challenge. The practitioner must acquire the needed skills during daily practice and by attending structured hands-on workshops whenever possible, in addition to using off-line software to gain more skill in volume manipulation. Various global organizations, at the forefront of which is the AIUM, through such initiatives as Ultrasound First (http://www.ultrasoundfirst.org), are raising awareness as to the tremendous role of ultrasound in general as a first-line imaging modality, and to 3D ultrasound in particular as an indispensible diagnostic tool in gynecology. Awareness will lead to better utilization and provide further clinical evidence, ultimately leading to better reimbursement. Volume sonography is here to stay despite all the obstacles. It is time to confidently incorporate it into daily clinical practice as a complementary modality to properly performed 2D sonography, and to maximize its potential role as an invaluable tool in helping the clinicians and families better appreciate complicated fetal anomalies. This will facilitate planning antepartum, intrapartum, and postpartum care. Caution must be exercised against its use for non-medical purposes. This novel method, when properly utilized, enhances the physician–patient relationship as well as patient-fetal bonding, while providing reassurance and valuable information as to the health and well-being of our future generations.

PRACTICAL PEARLS

- Even though reimbursement is limited, the practitioner should practice his 3D skills at every opportunity
- One must be very familiar with coding and the indications
- Caution is warranted against the non-medical use of ultrasound
- If possible, after a proper obstetrical examination, keep-sake images of the fetus help enhance the patient–physician relationship as well as patient–fetal bonding

References

Abuhamad AZ. 2004. Automated multiplanar imaging a novel approach to ultrasonography. *J Ultrasound Med* 23:573–576.

Abuhamad AZ. 2005. Standardization of 3-dimensional volumes in obstetric sonography: a required step for training and automation. *J Ultrasound Med* 24:397–401.

Abuhamad AZ. 2006. Clinical implications of the echo enhancement artifact in volume sonography of the uterus. *J Ultrasound Med* 25:1431–1435.

Abuhamad AZ, Singleton S, Zhao Y, Bocca S. 2006. The Z technique: an easy approach to the display of the midcoronal plane of the uterus in volume sonography. *J Ultrasound Med* 25:607–612.

Abuhamad AZ, Falkensammer P, Zhao Y. 2007. Automated sonography: defining the spatial relationships of standard diagnostic fetal cardiac planes in the second trimester of pregnancy. *J Ultrasound Med* 26:501–507.

Abu-Rustum, RS. NIPT: A Matter of Critical Timing. Prenatal Perspectives 2014; 2(2):5-6.

Abu-Rustum RS, Adra AM. 2007. Three-dimensional sonographic diagnosis of conjoined twins with fetal death in the first trimester. *J. Ultrasound Med* 27:1662–1663.

Abu-Rustum RS, Chaaban M. 2009. Is 3-dimensional sonography useful in the prenatal diagnosis of ambiguous genitalia? *J Ultrasound Med* 28:95–97.

Abu-Rustum RS, Ziade MF, Abu-Rustum SE. 2012. Defining the spatial relationships between 8 anatomic planes in the 11+6–13+6 week fetus. *Prenat Diagn* 32:875-882.

Abu-Rustum RS, Frangieh A, Fahed R, Soutou B, Abdelahad A. 2013. Limitations of 3-dimensional sonography in the prenatal evaluation of a skin denudation syndrome. *J Ultrasound Med* 32:1301–1303.

Achiron R, Gindes L, Zalel Y, Lipitz S, Weisz B. 2008. Three- and four-dimensional ultrasound: new methods for evaluating fetal thoracic anomalies. *Ultrasound Obstet Gynecol* 32:36–43.

ACOG Committee Opinion. 2004. Nonmedical use of obstetrical sonography. Number 297.

AIUM Press Release. 2002. AIUM Opposes Use of Ultrasound for Entertainment. www.aium.org/press/viewRelease.aspx?id=61

AIUM Press Release. 2004. The AIUM Reaffirms Its Opposition to Entertainment Ultrasound. www.aium.org/press/viewRelease.aspx?id = 66

AIUM Press Release. 2005a. Beyond Tom Cruise—The Bigger Ultrasound Picture. www.aium.org/press/viewRelease.aspx?id = 85

AIUM Press Release. 2005b. The AIUM Releases New Statement Regarding Keepsake Imaging. www.aium.org/press/viewRelease.aspx?id = 102

AIUM Press Release. 2005c. AIUM Discourages the Sale and Use of Ultrasound Equipment for Personal Use in the Home. www.aium.org/press/viewRelease.aspx?id = 114

AIUM Press Release. 2012. Keepsake Fetal Imaging. Approved April 1, 2012.

AIUM 76811 Task Force. 2014. Consensus report on the detailed fetal anatomical ultrasound examination: indications, components and qualifications. *J Ultrasound Med* 33:189–195.

Allen LM, Maestri MJ. 2008. Three-dimensional sonographic findings associated with ectrodactyly–ectodermal dysplasia–clefting syndrome. *J Ultrasound Med* 27:149–154.

Allen LM, Silverman RK, Nosovitch JT, Lohnes TM, Williams KD. 2008. Exploring 3-dimensional imaging techniques in the prenatal interrogation of cebocephaly. *J Ultrasound Med* 27:983–988.

Anandakumar C, Nuruddin Badruddin M, Chua TM, Wong YC, Chia D. 2002. First-trimester prenatal diagnosis of omphalocele using three-dimensional ultrasonography. *Ultrasound Obstet Gynecol* 20:635–636.

Antsaklis A, Daskalakis G, Theodora M, Hiridis P, Komita O, Blanas K, Anastaskis A. 2011. Assessment of nuchal translucency thickness and the fetal anatomy in the first trimester of pregnancy by two- and three-dimensional ultrasonography: a pilot study. *J Perinatal Med* 39:185–193.

APS Medical Billing. 2013. 3D Reconstruction. www.apsmedbill.com/newsletters/2013-02/3d-reconstruction.

Bahlmann F. 2000. Three-dimensional color power angiography of an aneurysm of the vein of Galen. *Ultrasound Obstet Gynecol* 15:341.

Bahmaie A, Hughes SW, Clark T, Milner A, Saunders J, Tilling K, Maxwell DJ. 2000. Serial fetal lung volume measurement using three-dimensional ultrasound. *Ultrasound Obstet Gynecol* 16:154–158.

Bault JP. 2006. Visualization of the fetal optic chiasma using three-dimensional ultrasound imaging. *Ultrasound Obstet Gynecol.* 28:862–864.

Benacerraf BR, Spiro R, Mitchell AG. 2000. Using three-dimensional ultrasound to detect craniosynostosis in a fetus with Pfeiffer syndrome. *Ultrasound Obstet Gynecol* 16:391–394.

Benacerraf BR, Benson CB, Abuhamad AZ, Copel JA, Abramowicz JS, DeVore GR, Doubilet PM, Lee W, Lev-Toaff AS, Merz E, Nelson TR, O'Neill MJ, Parsons AK, Platt LD, Pretorius DH, Timor-Tritsch IE. 2005. Three- and 4-dimensional ultrasound in obstetrics and gynecology. Proceedings of the American Institute of Ultrasound in Medicine Consensus Conference. *J Ulrasound Med* 24:1587–1597.

Benacerraf BR, Sadow PM, Barnewolt CE, Estroff JA, Benson C. 2006. Cleft of the secondary palate without cleft lip diagnosed with three-dimensional ultrasound and magnetic resonance imaging in a fetus with Fryns' syndrome. *Ultrasound Obstet Gynecol* 27:566–570.

Benacerraf BR. 2008. *Ultrasound of Fetal Syndromes*. Second Edition. London: Churchill Livingstone.

Benavides-Serralde A, Hernández-Andrade E, Fernández-Delgado J, Plasencia W, Scheier M, Crispi F, Figueras F, Nicolaides KH, Gratacós E. 2009. Three-dimensional sonographic calculation of the volume of intracranial structures in growth-restricted and appropriate-for-gestational age fetuses. *Ultrasound Obstet Gynecol* 33:530–537.

Benoit B. 1999. Three-dimensional ultrasonography of congenital ichthyosis. *Ultrasound Obstet Gynecol* 13:380.

Benoit B, Chaoui R. 2005. Three-dimensional ultrasound with maximal mode rendering: a novel technique for the diagnosis of bilateral or unilateral absence or hypoplasia of nasal bones in second-trimester screening for Down syndrome. *Ultrasound Obstet Gynecol* 25:19–24.

Bharudi M, Fong K, Toi A, Tomlinson G, Okun N. 2010. Fetal anatomic survey using three-dimensional ultrasound in conjunction with first-trimester nuchal translucency screening. *Prenat Diagn* 30:267–273.

Blaas HG, Eik-Nes SH, Berg TKS, Olstad BAB. 1995. Three-dimensional imaging of the brain cavities in human embryos. *Ultrasound Obstet Gynecol* 5:228–232.

Blaas HGK, Eik-Nes SH, Isaksen CV. 2000a.The detection of spina bifida before 10 gestational weeks using two- and three-dimensional ultrasound. *Ultrasound Obstet Gynecol* 16:25–29.

Blaas HGK, Eik-Nes SH, Vainio T, Vogt Isaksen C. 2000b. Alobar holoprosencephaly at 9 weeks gestational age visualized by two- and three-dimensional ultrasound. *Ultrasound Obstet Gynecol* 15:62–65.

Blaicher W, Lee A, Deutinger J, Bernaschek G. 2001. Sirenomelia: early prenatal diagnosis with combined two- and three-dimensional sonography. *Ultrasound Obstet Gynecol* 17:542–543.

Bocca SM, Oehninger S, Stadtmauer L, Agard J, Duran EH, Sarhan A, Horton S, Abuhamad AZ. 2012. A study of the cost, accuracy, and benefits of 3-dimensional sonography compared with hysterosalpingography in women with uterine abnormalities. *J Ultrasound Med* 31:81–85.

Bocca SM, Abuhamad AZ. 2013. Use of 3-dimensional sonography to assess uterine anomalies. *J Ultrasound Med* 32:1–6.

Bongain A, Benoit B, Ejnes L, Lambert JC, Gillet JY. 2002. Harlequin fetus: three-dimensional sonographic findings and new diagnostic approach. *Ultrasound Obstet Gynecol* 20:82–85.

Bonilla-Musoles F, Raga F, Villalobos A, Blanes J, Osborne NG. 1998. First-trimester neck abnormalities: three-dimensional evaluation. *J Ultrasound Med* 17:419–425.

Bonilla-Musoles F, Machado LE, Bailão LA, Osborne NG, Raga F. 2001. Abdominal wall defects two- versus three-dimensional ultrasonographic diagnosis. *J Ultrasound Med* 20:379–389.

Bonilia-Musoles F, Machado LE, Raga F, Osborne NG, Bonilla Jr F. 2002. Prenatal diagnosis of sacrococcygeal teratomas by two- and three-dimensional ultrasound. *Ultrasound Obstet Gynecol* 19:200–205.

Borrell A, Santolaya-Forgas J, Horbaczewski C, Henry R, Dunn-Albanese L, Robinson JN. 2011. Is the starting section for 3D volume acquisition in the first trimester relevant in the post hoc analysis of aneuploidy screening markers and fetal anatomy? *Prenat Diagn* 31:1305–1310.

Bromley B, Shipp TD, Benacerraf BR. 2010. Structural anomalies in early embryonic death: a 3-dimensional pictorial essay. *J Ultrasound Med* 29:445–453.

Budorick NE, Pretorius DH, Johnson DD, Nelson TR, Tartar MK, Lou KV. 1998. Three-dimensional ultrasonography of the fetal distal lower extremity: normal and abnormal. *J Ultrasound Med* 17:649–660.

Cafici D, Iglesias A. 2002. Prenatal diagnosis of severe hypospadias with two- and three-dimensional sonography. *J Ultrasound Med* 21:1423–1426.

Campbell S, Lees CC. 2003. The three-dimensional reverse face (3D RF) view for the diagnosis of cleft palate. *Ultrasound Obstet Gynecol* 22:552–554.

Campbell S, Lees C, Moscoso G, Hall P. 2005. Ultrasound antenatal diagnosis of cleft palate by a new technique: the 3D "reverse face" view. *Ultrasound Obstet Gynecol* 25:12–18.

Chaoui R, Zodan-Marin T, Wisser J. 2002. Marked splenomegaly in fetal cytomegalovirus infection: detection supported by three-dimensional power Doppler ultrasound. *Ultrasound Obstet Gynecol* 20:299–302.

Chaoui R, Hoffmann J, Heling KS. 2004. Three-dimensional (3D) and 4D color Doppler fetal echocardiography using spatio-temporal image correlation (STIC). *Ultrasound Obstet Gynecol* 23:535–545.

Chaoui R, Levaillant JM, Benoit B, Faro C, Wegrzyn P, Nicolaides KH. 2005. Three-dimensional sonographic description of abnormal metopic suture in second- and third-trimester fetuses. *Ultrasound Obstet Gynecol* 26:761–764.

Correa FF, Lara C, Bellver J, Remohí J, Pellicer A, Serra V. 2006. Examination of the fetal brain by transabdominal three-dimensional ultrasound: potential for routine neurosonographic studies. *Ultrasound Obstet Gynecol* 27:503–508.

Dagklis T, Borenstein M, Peralta CFA, Faro C, Nicolaides KH. 2006. Three-dimensional evaluation of mid-facial hypoplasia in fetuses with trisomy 21 at 11 + 0 to 13 + 6 weeks of gestation. *Ultrasound Obstet Gynecol* 28:261–265.

Devonald KJ, Ellwood DA, Griffiths KA, Kossoff G, Gill RW, Kadi AP, Nash DM, Warren PS, Davis W, Picker R. 1995. Volume imaging: three-dimenional appreciation of the fetal head and face. *J Ultrasound Med* 14:919–925.

DeVore GR, Falkensammer P, Sklansky MS, Platt LD. 2003. Spatio-temporal image correlation (STIC): new technology for evaluation of the fetal heart. *Ultrasound Obstet Gynecol* 22:380–387.

DeVore GR, Polanco B, Sklansky MS, Platt LD. 2004. The "spin" technique: a new method for examination of the fetal outflow tracts using three-dimensional ultrasound. *Ultrasound Obstet Gynecol* 24:72–82.

Dikkeboom CM, Roelfsema NM, van Adrichem LNA, Wladimiroff JW. 2004. The role of three-dimensional ultrasound in visualizing the fetal cranial sutures and fontanels during the second half of pregnancy. *Ultrasound Obstet Gynecol* 24:412–416.

Duin LK, Willekes C, Vossen M, Beckers M, Offermans J, Nijhuis JG. 2008. Reproducibility of fetal renal pelvis volume measurement using three-dimensional ultrasound. *Ultrasound Obstetrics Gynecol* 31:657–661.

Dulay AT, Schwartz N, Laser A, Greco MA, Monteagudo A, Timor-Tritsch IE. 2006. Two- and 3-dimensional sonographic diagnosis of a vesicorectal fistula in cloacal dysgenesis sequence. *J Ultrasound Med* 25:1489–1494.

Espinoza J, Lee W, Comstock C, Romero R, Yeo L, Rizzo G, Paladini D, Viñals F, Achiron R, Gindes L, Abuhamad A, Sinkovskaya E, Russell E, Yagel S. 2010. Collaborative study on 4-dimensional echocardiography for the diagnosis of fetal heart defects: the COFEHD study. *J Ultrasound Med* 29:1573–1580.

Faro C, Benoit B, Wegrzyn P, Chaoui R, Nicolaides KH. 2005. Three-dimensional sonographic description of the fetal frontal bones and metopic suture. *Ultrasound Obstet Gynecol* 26:618–621.

Fauchon DEV, Benzie RJ, Wye DA, Cairns DR. 2008. What information on fetal anatomy can be provided by a single first-trimester transabdominal three-dimensional sweep? *Ultrasound Obstet Gynecol* 31:266–270.

Faure JM, Captier G, Bäumler M, Boulot P. 2007. Sonographic assessment of normal fetal palate using three-dimensional imaging: a new technique. *Ultrasound Obstet Gynecol* 29:159–165.

Faure JM, Bäumler M, Boulot P, Bigorre M, Captier G. 2008. Prenatal assessment of the normal fetal soft palate by three-dimensional ultrasound examination: is there an objective technique? *Ultrasound Obstet Gynecol* 31:652–656.

Gagel K, Heling KS, Kalache KD, Chaoui R. 2003. Prenatal diagnosis of an intracranial arteriovenous fistula in the posterior fossa on the basis of color and three-dimensional power Doppler ultrasonography. *J Ultrasound Med* 22:1399–1403.

GE Healthcare. 2011. Reimbursement information for diagnostic ultrasound procedures completed by obstetricians. www3.gehealthcare.com/en/Products/Categories/~/media/Downloads/us/Product/Product-Categories/Ultrasound/GEHealthcare-Brochure_Reimbursement-Info-Obstetricians.pdf

Gerards FA, Engels MAJ, Barkhof F, van den Dungen FAM, Vermeulen RJ, van Vugt JMG. 2003. Prenatal diagnosis of aneurysms of the vein of Galen (vena magna cerebri) with conventional sonography, three-dimensional sonography, and magnetic resonance imaging. Report of 2 cases. *J Ultrasound Med* 22:1363–1368.

Gerards FA, Engels MAJ, Twisk JWR, van Vugt JMG. 2006. Normal fetal lung volume measured with three-dimensional ultrasound. *Ultrasound Obstet Gynecol* 27:134–144.

Gerards FA, Twisk JWR, Bakker M, Barkhof F, van Vugt JMG. 2007. Fetal lung volume: three-dimensional ultrasonography compared with magnetic resonance imaging. *Ultrasound Obstet Gynecol* 29:533–536.

Ghi T, Contro E, Farina A, Nobile M, Pilu G. 2010. Three-dimensional ultrasound in monitoring progression of labor: a reproducibility study. *Ultrasound Obstet Gynecol* 36:500–506.

Gindes L, Benoit B, Pretorius DH, Achiron R. 2008. Abnormal number of fetal ribs on 3-dimensional ultrasonography associated anomalies and outcomes in 75 fetuses. *J Ultrasound Med* 27:1263–1271.

Gindes L, Hegesh J, Weisz B, Gilboa Y, Achiron R. 2009. Three and four dimensional ultrasound: a novel method for evaluating fetal cardiac anomalies. *Prenat Diagn* 29:645–653.

Glanc P, Umranikar S, Koff D, Tomlinson G, Chitayat D. 2007. Fetal sex assignment by sonographic evaluation of the pelvic organs in the second and third trimesters of pregnancy. *J Ultrasound Med* 26:563–569.

Greene N, Platt LD. 2005. Nonmedical use of ultrasound: greater harm than good? *J Ultrasound Med* 2:123–125.

Hamill N, Yeo L, Romero R, Hassan SS, Myers SA, Mittal P, Kusanovic JP, Balasubramaniam M, Chaiworapongsa T, Vaisbuch E, Espinoza J, Gotsch F, Goncalves LF, Lee W. 2011. Fetal cardiac ventricular volume, cardiac output, and ejection fraction determined with 4-dimensional ultrasound using spatiotemporal image correlation and virtual organ computer-aided analysis. *Am J Obstet Gynecol* 205:76.e1–10.

Hata T, Aoki S, Manabe A, Hata K, Miyazaki K. 1998a. Visualization of fetal genitalia by three-dimensional ultrasonography in the second and third trimesters. *J Ultrasound Med* 17:137–139.

Hata T, Aoki S, Akiyama M, Yanagihara T, Miyazaki K. 1998b. Three-dimensional ultrasonographic assessment of fetal hands and feet. *Ultrasound Obstet Gynecol* 12:235–239.

Heling KS, Chaoui R, Bollmann R. 2000. Prenatal diagnosis of an aneurysm of the vein of Galen with three-dimensional color power angiography. *Ultrasound Obstet Gynecol* 15:333–336.

Hoffman JIE, Christianson R. 1978. Congenital heart disease in a cohort of 19502 births with long-term follow-up. *Am J Cardiol* 42:641–647.

Hsu CY, Chen CP, Lin CJ. 2007. An aberrant renal artery arising from the iliac artery imaged by three-dimensional power Doppler ultrasonography: a sign of fetal horseshoe kidney. *Ultrasound Obstet Gynecol* 29:358–359.

Hsu TY, Hsu JJ, Chang SY, Chang MS. 2002. Prenatal three-dimensional sonographic images associated with Treacher Collins syndrome. *Ultrasound Obstet Gynecol* 19:413–414.

Hull AD, Pretorius DH, Lev-Toaff A, Budorick NE, Salerno CC, Johnson MM, James G, Nelson TR. 2000. Artifacts and the visualization of fetal distal extremities using three-dimensional ultrasound. *Ultrasound Obstet Gynecol* 16:341–344.

Hunter S, Heads A, Wyllie J, Robson S. 2000. Prenatal diagnosis of congenital heart disease in the northern region of England: benefits of a training programme for obstetric ultrasonographers. *Heart* 84:294–298.

Izquierdo MT, Bahamonde A, Domene J. 2009. Prenatal diagnosis of a complete cleft sternum with 3-dimensional sonography. *J Ultrasound Med* 28:379–383.

Johnson JM, Benoit B, Pierre-Louis J, Keating S, Chitayat D. 2005. Early prenatal diagnosis of oculoauriculofrontonasal syndrome by three-dimensional ultrasound. *Ultrasound Obstet Gynecol* 25:184–186.

Jouannic JM, Rosenblatt J, Demaria F, Jacobs R, Aubry MC, Benifla JL. 2005. Contribution of three-dimensional volume contrast imaging to the sonographic assessment of the fetal uterus. *Ultrasound Obstet Gynecol* 26:567–570.

Kalache KD, Espinoza J, Chaiworapongsa T, Londono J, Schoen ML, Treadwell MC, Lee W, Romero R. 2003. Three-dimensional ultrasound fetal lung volume measurement: a systematic study comparing the multiplanar method with the rotational (VOCAL) technique. *Ultrasound Obstet Gynecol* 21:111–118.

Khandelwal M, Silva J, Chan L, Reece EA. 1999. Three-dimensional ultrasonographic technology to assess and compare echodensity of fetal bowel, bone, and liver in the second trimester of pregnancy. *J Ultrasound Med* 18:691–695.

Kim MS, Jeanty P, Turner C, Benoit B. 2008. Three-dimensional sonographic evaluations of embryonic brain development. *J Ultrasound Med* 27:119–124.

Krakow D, Santulli T, Platt LD. 2001. Use of three-dimensional ultrasonography in differentiating craniosynostosis from severe fetal molding. *J Ultrasound Med* 20:427–431.

Krakow D, Williams III J, Poehl M, Rimoin DL, Platt LD. 2003. Use of three-dimensional ultrasound imaging in the diagnosis of prenatal-onset skeletal dysplasias. *Ultrasound Obstet Gynecol* 21:467–472.

Kuno A, Hayashi Y, Akiyama M, Yamashiro C, Tanaka H, Yanagihara T, Hata T. 2002. Three-dimensional sonographic measurement of liver volume in the small-for-gestational-age fetus. *J Ultrasound Med* 21:361–366.

Kurjak A, Abo-Yaqoub S, Stanojevic M, Basgul Yigiter A, Vasilj O, Lebit D, Naim Shaddad A, Badreldeen A, Nese Kavak Z, Miskovic B, Vladareanu R, Spalldi Barisic L, Azumendi G, Younis M, Pooh RK, Salihagic Kadic A. 2010. The potential of 4D sonography in the assessment of fetal neurobehavior—multicentric study in high-risk pregnancies. *J Perinat Med* 38:77–82.

Laudy JAM, Janssen MMM, Struyk PC, Stijnen T, Wallenburg HCS, Wladimiroff JW. 1998. Fetal liver volume measurement by three-dimensional ultrasonography: a preliminary study. *Ultrasound Obstet Gynecol* 12:93–96.

Lee A, Kratochwil A, Deutinger J, Bernaschek G. 1995. Three-dimensional ultrasound in diagnosing phocomelia. *Ultrasound Obstet Gynecol* 5:238–240.

Lee SM, Park SK, Shim SS, Jun JK, Park JS, Syn HC. 2007. Measurement of fetal urine production by three-dimensional ultrasonography in normal pregnancy. *Ultrasound Obstet Gynecol* 30:281–286.

Lee TH, Shih JC, Peng SSF, Lee CN, Shyu MK, Hsieh FJ. 2000. Prenatal depiction of angioarchitecture of an aneurysm of the vein of Galen with three-dimensional color power angiography. *Ultrasound Obstet Gynecol* 15:337–340.

Lee W, Blanckaert K, Bronsteen RA, Huang R, Romero R. 2001a. Fetal iliac angle measurements by three-dimensional sonography. *Ultrasound Obstet Gynecol* 18:150–154.

Lee W, Deter RL, Ebersole JD, Huang R, Blanckaert K, Romero R. 2001b. Birth weight prediction by three-dimensional ultrasonography fractional limb volume. *J Ultrasound Med* 20:1283–1292.

Lee W, Chaiworapongsa T, Romero R, Williams R, McNie B, Johnson A, Treadwell M, Comstock CH. 2002a. A diagnostic approach for the evaluation of spina bifida by three-dimensional ultrasonography. *J Ultrasound Med* 21:619–626.

Lee W, McNie B, Chaiworapongsa T, Conoscenti G, Kalache KD, Vettraino IM, Romero R, Comstock CH. 2002b. Three-dimensional ultrasonographic presentation of micrognathia. *J Ultrasound Med* 21:775–781.

Lee W, Deter RL, McNie B, Gonçalves LF, Espinoza J, Chaiworapongsa T, Romero R. 2004. Individualized growth assessment of fetal soft tissue using fractional thigh volume. *Ultrasound Obstet Gynecol* 24:766–774.

Lee W, Balasubramaniam M, Deter RL, Hassan SS, Gotsch F, Kusanovic JP, Gonçalves LF, Romero R. 2009. Fractional limb volume—a soft tissue parameter of fetal body composition: validation, technical considerations and normal ranges during pregnancy. *Ultrasound Obstet Gynecol* 33:427–440.

Levaillant JM, Mabille M. 2005. Fetal sphenoid bone: imaging using three-dimensional ultrasound and computed tomography. *Ultrasound Obstet Gynecol* 31:229–231.

Lev-Toaff AS, Ozhan S, Pretorius D, Bega G, Kurtz AB, Kuhlman K. 2000. Three-dimensional multiplanar ultrasound for fetal gender assignment: value of the mid-sagittal plane. *Ultrasound Obstet Gynecol* 16:345–350.

Lin HH, Liang RI, Chang FM, Chang CH, Yu CH, Yang HB. 1998. Prenatal diagnosis of otocephaly using two-dimensional and three-dimensional ultrasonography. *Ultrasound Obstet Gynecol* 11:361–363.

Loureiro T, Cunha M, Jesus JM, Beires J, Montenegro N. 2008. Congenital abdominal hemangioma: three-dimensional power Doppler imaging and volume acquisition in the assessment of tumor vasculature. *Ultrasound Obstet Gynecol* 31:593–596.

Malinger G, Lerman-Sagie T, Viñals F. 2006. Three-dimensional sagittal reconstruction of the corpus callosum: fact or artifact? *Ultrasound Obstet Gynecol* 28:742–743.

Martínez Ten P, Pérez Pedregosa J, Santacruz B, Adiego B, Barrón E, Sepúlveda W. 2009. Three-dimensional ultrasound diagnosis of cleft palate: "reverse face," "flipped face" or "oblique face"—which method is best? *Ultrasound Obstet Gynecol* 33:399–406.

Matsumi H, Kozuma S, Baba K, Kobayashi K, Yoshikawa H, Okai T, Taketani Y. 1996. Three-dimensional ultrasound is useful in diagnosing the fetus with abdominal wall defect. *Ultrasound Obstet Gynecol* 8:356–358.

McGahan MC, Ramos GA, Landry C, Wolfson T, Sowell BB, D'Agostini D, Patino C, Nelson TR, Pretorius DH. 2008. Multislice display of the fetal face using 3-dimensional ultrasonography. *J Ultrasound Med* 27:1573–1581.

Merhi ZO, Haberman S, Roberts J, Gretta Sobol-Benin G. 2005. Prenatal diagnosis of palatal teratoma by 3-dimensional sonography and color Doppler imaging. *J Ultrasound Med* 24:1317–1320.

Merz E, Weber G, Bahlmann F, Miric-Tesanic D. 1997. Application of transvaginal and abdominal three-dimensional ultrasound for the detection or exclusion of malformations of the fetal face. *Ultrasound Obstet Gynecol* 9:237–243.

Merz E. 1998. Three dimensional ultrasound—a requirement for prenatal diagnosis? *Ultrasound Obstet Gynecol* 12:225–226.

Merz E, Miric-Tesanic D, Bahlmann F, Sedlaczek H. 1999. Prenatal diagnosis of fetal ambiguous gender using three-dimensional sonography. *Ultrasound Obstet Gynecol* 13:217–219.

Michailidis GD, Papageorgiou P, Economides D. 2002. Assessment of fetal anatomy in the first trimester using two- and three-dimensional ultrasound. *Br J Radiol* 75:215–219.

Mittal P, Gonçalves LF, Kusanovic JP, Espinoza J, Lee W, Nien JK, Eleazar Soto E, Romero R. 2007. Objective evaluation of Sylvian fissure development by multiplanar 3-dimensional ultrasonography. *J Ultrasound Med* 26:347–353.

Moeglin D, Benoit B. 2001. Three-dimensional sonographic aspects in the antenatal diagnosis of achondroplasia. *Ultrasound Obstet Gynecol* 18:81–83.

Moeglin D, Talmant C, Duyme M, Lopez AC. 2005. Fetal lung volumetry using two- and three-dimensional ultrasound. *Ultrasound Obstet Gynecol* 25:119–127.

Molina FS, Faro C, Sotiriadis A, Dagklis T, Nicolaides KH. 2008. Heart stroke volume and cardiac output by four-dimensional ultrasound in normal fetuses. *Ultrasound Obstet Gynecol* 32:181–187.

Monteagudo A, Mayberry P, Rebarber A, Paidas M, Timor-Tritsch IE. 2002. Sirenomelia sequence first-trimester diagnosis with both two- and three-dimensional sonography. *J Ultrasound Med* 21:915–920.

Muench MV, Zheng M, Bilica PM, Canterino JC. 2008. Prenatal diagnosis of a fetal epidural hematoma using 2- and 3-dimensional sonography and magnetic resonance imaging. *J Ultrasound Med* 27:1369–1373.

Nath CA, Oyelese Y, Yeo L, Chavez M, Kontopoulos EV, Giannina G, Smulian JC, Vintzileos AM. 2005. Three-dimensional sonography in the evaluation and management of fetal goiter. *Ultrasound Obstet Gynecol* 25:312–314.

Naylor CS, Carlson DE, Santulli, Jr, T, Platt, LD. 2001. Use of three-dimensional ultrasonography for prenatal diagnosis of ambiguous genitalia. *J Ultrasound Med* 20:1365–1367.

Nelson TR, Pretorius DH, Hull A, Riccabona M, Sklansky MS, James G. 2000. Sources and impact of artifacts on clinical three-dimensional ultrasound imaging. *Ultrasound Obstet Gynecol* 16:374–383.

Osada H, Iitsuka Y, Masuda K, Sakamoto R, Kaku K, Seki K, Sekiya S. 2002. Application of lung volume measurement by three-dimensional ultrasonography for clinical assessment of fetal lung development. *J Ultrasound Med* 21:841–847.

Pagani G, Palai N, Zatti S, Fratelli N, Prefumo F, Frusca T. 2014. Fetal weight estimation in gestational diabetic pregnancies: comparison between conventional and three-dimensional fractional thigh volume methods using gestation-adjusted projection. *Ultrasound Obstet Gynecol* 43:72–76.

Paladini D, Vassallo M, Sglavo G, Lapadula C, Longo M, Nappi C. 2005. Cavernous lymphangioma of the face and neck: prenatal diagnosis by three-dimensional ultrasound. *Ultrasound Obstet Gynecol* 26:300–302.

Paladini D, Volpe P. 2006. Posterior fossa and vermian morphometry in the characterization of fetal cerebellar abnormalities: a prospective three-dimensional ultrasound study. *Ultrasound Obstet Gynecol* 27:482–489.

Paladini D, Sglavo G, Penner I, Pastore G, Nappi C. 2007. Fetuses with Down syndrome have an enlarged anterior fontanelle in the second trimester of pregnancy. *Ultrasound Obstet Gynecol* 30:824–829.

Paladini D, Vassallo M, Sglavo G, Pastore G, Lapadula C, Nappi C. 2008a. Normal and abnormal development of the fetal anterior fontanelle: a three-dimensional ultrasound study. *Ultrasound Obstet Gynecol* 32:755–761.

Paladini D, Sglavo G, Greco E, Nappi C. 2008b. Cardiac screening by STIC: can sonologists performing the 20-week anomaly scan pick up outflow tract abnormalities by scrolling the A-plane of STIC volumes? *Ultrasound Obstet Gynecol* 32:865–870.

Paris L, Cabaret AS, Grall JY. 2004. Three-dimensional imaging of the portal sinus anatomy. *Ultrasound Obstet Gynecol* 23:207–208.

Peralta CFA, Falcon O, Wegrzyn P, Faro C, Nicolaides KH. 2005. Assessment of the gap between the fetal nasal bones at 11 to 13 + 6 weeks of gestation by three-dimensional ultrasound. *Ultrasound Obstet Gynecol* 25:464–467.

Peralta CFA, Kazan-Tannus JF, Bunduki V, Santos EM, de Castrom C, Cerri GG, Zugaib M. 2006a. Evaluation of the agreement between 3-dimensional ultrasonography and magnetic resonance imaging for fetal lung volume measurement. *J Ultrasound Med* 25:461–467.

Peralta CFA, Cavoretto P, Csapo B, Falcon O, Nicolaides KH. 2006b. Lung and heart volumes by three-dimensional ultrasound in normal fetuses at 12–32 weeks' gestation. *Ultrasound Obstet Gynecol* 27:128–133.

Pilu G, Visentin A, Ambrosini G, D'Antona D, Andrisani A. 2005. Three-dimensional sonography of unilateral Tessier number 7 cleft in a mid-trimester fetus. *Ultrasound Obstet Gynecol* 26:98–99.

Pilu G, Segata M, Ghi T, Carletti A, Perolo A, Santini D, Bonasoni P, Tani G, Rizzo N. 2006. Diagnosis of midline anomalies of the fetal brain with the three-dimensional median view. *Ultrasound Obstet Gynecol* 27:522–529.

Pilu G, Segata M. 2007. A novel technique for visualization of the normal and cleft fetal secondary palate: angled insonation and three-dimensional ultrasound. *Ultrasound Obstet Gynecol* 29:166–169.

Plasencia W, Dagklis T, Borenstein M, Csapo B, Nicolaides KH. 2007. Assessment of the corpus callosum at 20–24 weeks' gestation by three-dimensional ultrasound examination. *Ultrasound Obstet Gynecol* 30:169–172.

Platt LD, DeVore GR, Pretorius DH. 2006. Improving cleft palate/cleft lip antenatal diagnosis by 3-dimensional sonography the "flipped face" view. *J Ultrasound Med* 25:1423–1430.

Pohls UG, Rempen A. 1998. Fetal lung volumetry by three-dimensional ultrasound. *Ultrasound Obstet Gynecol* 11:6–12.

Ramón y Cajal CL, Ocampo Martínez R. 2003. Prenatal diagnosis of duodenal atresia with three-dimensional sonography. *Ultrasound Obstet Gynecol* 22:656–657.

Ramón y Cajal CL, Martínez RO. 2005. Prenatal observation of fetal defecation using four-dimensional ultrasonography. *Ultrasound Obstet Gynecol* 26:794–795.

Rembouskos G, Cicero S, Longo D, Vandecruys H, Nicolaides KH. 2004. Assessment of the fetal nasal bone at 11–14 weeks of gestation by three-dimensional ultrasound. *Ultrasound Obstet Gynecol* 23:232–236.

Rizzo G, Capponi A, Muscatello A, Cavicchioni O, Vendola M, Arduini D. 2008. Examination of the fetal heart by four-dimensional ultrasound with spatio temporal image correlation during routine second-trimester examination: the "three-steps technique." *Fetal Diagn Ther* 24:126–131.

Rochelson B, Vohra N, Krantz D, Macri VJ. 2006. Geometric morphometric analysis of shape outlines of the normal and abnormal fetal skull using three-dimensional sonographic multiplanar display. *Ultrasound Obstet Gynecol* 27:167–172.

Roelfsema NM, Hop WCJ, Wladimiroff JW. 2006. Three-dimensional sonographic determination of normal fetal mandibular and maxillary size during the second half of pregnancy. *Ultrasound Obstet Gynecol* 28:950–957.

Roelfsema NM, Hop HCJ, van Adrichem LNA, Wladimiroff JW. 2007a. Craniofacial variability index in utero: a three-dimensional ultrasound study. *Ultrasound Obstet Gynecol* 29:258–264.

Roelfsema NM, Hop WCJ, van Adrichem LNA, Wladimiroff JW. 2007b. Craniofacial variability index determined by three-dimensional ultrasound in isolated vs. syndromal fetal cleft lip/palate. *Ultrasound Obstet Gynecol* 29:265–270.

Roelfsema NM, Grijseels EWM, Hop WCJ, Wladimiroff JW. 2007c. Three-dimensional sonography of prenatal skull base development. *Ultrasound Obstet Gynecol* 29:372–377.

Roman AS, Monteagudo A, Timor-Tritsch I, Rebarber A. 2004. First-trimester diagnosis of sacrococcygeal teratoma: the role of three-dimensional ultrasound. *Ultrasound Obstet Gynecol* 23:612–614.

Rotten D, Levaillant JM. 2004a.Two- and three-dimensional sonographic assessment of the fetal face. A systematic analysis of the normal face. *Ultrasound Obstet Gynecol* 23:224–231.

Rotten D, Levaillant JM. 2004b. Two- and three-dimensional sonographic assessment of the fetal face. 2. Analysis of cleft lip, alveolus and palate. *Ultrasound Obstet Gynecol* 24:402–411.

Ruano R, Dumez Y, Dommergues M. 2003a. Three-dimensional ultrasonographic appearance of the fetal akinesia deformation sequence. *J Ultrasound Med* 22:593–599.

Ruano R, Benachi A, Aubry MC, Brunelle F, Dumez Y, Dommergues M. 2003b. Perinatal three-dimensional color power Doppler ultrasonography of vein of Galen aneurysms. *J Ultrasound Med* 22:1357–1362.

Ruano R, Joubin L, Sonigo P, Benachi A, Aubry, Thalabard JC, Brunelle F, Dumezm Y, Dommergues M. 2004. Fetal lung volume estimated by 3-dimensional ultrasonography and magnetic resonance imaging in cases with isolated congenital diaphragmatic hernia. *J Ultrasound Med* 23:353–358.

Ruano R, Benachi A, Aubry M, Dumez Y, Dommergues M. 2004a. Volume contrast imaging: a new approach to identify fetal thoracic structures. *J Ultrasound Med* 23:403–408.

Ruano R, Molho M, Roume J, Ville Y. 2004b. Prenatal diagnosis of fetal skeletal dysplasias by combining two-dimensional and three-dimensional ultrasound and intrauterine three-dimensional helical computer tomography. *Ultrasound Obstet Gynecol* 24:134–140.

Ruano R, Martinovic J, Dommergues M, Aubry MC, Dumez Y, Benachi A. 2005a. Accuracy of fetal lung volume assessed by three-dimensional sonography. *Ultrasound Obstet Gynecol* 26:725–730.

Ruano R, Benachi A, Aubry MC, Revillon Y, Emond S, Dumez Y, Dommergues M. 2005b. Prenatal diagnosis of pulmonary sequestration using three-dimensional power Doppler ultrasound. *Ultrasound Obstet Gynecol* 25:128–133.

Ruano R, Joubin L, Aubry MC, Thalabard JC, Dommergues, M, Dumez Y, Benachi A. 2006. A nomogram of fetal lung volumes estimated by 3-dimensional ultrasonography using the rotational technique (virtual organ computer-aided analysis). *J Ultrasound Med* 25:701–709.

Ruano R, Takashi E, Schultz R, Zugaib M. 2008. Prenatal diagnosis of posterior mediastinal lymphangioma by two- and three-dimensional ultrasonography. *Ultrasound Obstet Gynecol* 31:697–700.

Ruano R, Pimenta EJ, Duarte S, Zugaib M. 2009. Four-dimensional ultrasonographic imaging of fetal lower urinary tract obstruction and guidance of percutaneous cystoscopy. *Ultrasound Obstet Gynecol* 33:250–252.

Sabogal JC, Becker E, Bega G, Komwilaisak R, Berghella V, Weiner S, Tolosa J. 2004. Reproducibility of fetal lung volume measurements with 3-dimensional ultrasonography. *J Ultrasound Med* 23:347–352.

Sakhel K, Benson CB, Platt LD, Goldstein SR, Benacerraf BB. 2013. Begin with the basics: role of 3-dimensional sonography as a first-line imaging technique in the cost-effective evaluation of gynecologic pelvic disease. *J Ultrasound Med* 32:381–388.

Sallout BI, D'Agostini DA, Pretorius DH. 2006. Prenatal diagnosis of spondylocostal dysostosis with 3-dimensional ultrasonography. *J Ultrasound Med* 25:539–543.

Sammour RRN, Leibovitz Z, Degani S, Ohel G. 2008. Prenatal diagnosis of small-bowel volvulus using 3-dimensional doppler sonography. *J Ultrasound Med* 27:1655–1661.

Schild RL, Wallny T, Fimmers R, Hansmann M. 1999. Fetal lumbar spine volumetry by three-dimensional ultrasound. *Ultrasound Obstet Gynecol* 13:335–339.

Schild RL, Plath H, Hofstaetter H, Hansmann M. 2000. Diagnosis of a fetal mesoblastic nephroma by 3D-ultrasound. *Ultrasound Obstet Gynecol* 15:533–536.

Sepulveda W, Sandoval R, Carstens E, Gutierrez J, Vasquez P. 2003. Hypohidrotic ectodermal dysplasia prenatal diagnosis by three-dimensional ultrasonography. *J Ultrasound Med* 22:731–735.

Sepulveda W, Sepulveda-Swatson E, Sanchez J. 2004. Diastrophic dysplasia: prenatal three-dimensional ultrasound findings. *Ultrasound Obstet Gynecol* 23:312–314.

Sepulveda W, Wojakowski AB, Elias D, Otaño L, Gutierrez J. 2005.Congenital dacryocystocele prenatal 2- and 3-dimensional sonographic findings. *J Ultrasound Med* 24:225–230.

Sepulveda W. 2007. Prenatal 3-dimensional sonographic depiction of the Wolf Hirschhorn phenotype. The "Greek Warrior Helmet" and "Tulip" signs. *J Ultrasound Med* 26:407–410.

Sepulveda W, Lutz I, Be C. 2007. Holoprosencephaly at 9 weeks 6 days in a triploid fetus two- and 3-dimensional sonographic findings. *J Ultrasound Med* 26:411–414.

Shaw L, Al-Malt A, Carlan SJ, Plumley D, Greenbaum L, Kosko J. 2004. Congenital epulis three-dimensional ultrasonographic findings and clinical implications. *J Ultrasound Med* 23:1121–1124.

Sherer DM, Zigalo A, Abulafia O. 2006. Prenatal 3-dimensional sonographic diagnosis of a massive fetal epignathus occluding the oral orifice and both nostrils at 35 weeks' gestation. *J Ultrasound Med* 25:1503–1505.

Shih JC, Hsu WC, Chou HC, Peng SS, Chen LK, Chang YL, Hsieh FJ. 2005. Prenatal three-dimensional ultrasound and magnetic resonance imaging evaluation of a fetal oral tumor in preparation for the ex-utero intrapartum treatment (EXIT) procedure. *Ultrasound Obstet Gynecol* 25:76–79.

Shipp TD, Mulliken JB, Bromley B, Benacerraf B. 2002. Three-dimensional prenatal diagnosis of frontonasal malformation and unilateral cleft lip/palate. *Ultrasound Obstet Gynecol* 20:290–293.

Simioni C, Nardozza LM, Araujo Júnior E, Rolo LC, Zamith M, Caetano AC, Moron AF. 2011. Heart stroke volume, cardiac output, and ejection fraction in 265 normal fetus in the second half of gestation assessed by 4D ultrasound using spatiotemporal image correlation. *J Matern Fetal Neonatal Med* 24:1159–1167.

Soto E, Richani K, Gonçalves LF, Devers P, Espinoza J, Lee W, Treadwell MC, Romero R. 2006. Three-dimensional ultrasound in the prenatal diagnosis of cleidocranial dysplasia associated with B-cell immunodeficiency. *Ultrasound Obstet Gynecol* 27:574–579.

Tanaka Y, Miyazaki T, Kanenishi K, Tanaka H, Yanagihara T, Hata T. 2002. Antenatal three-dimensional sonographic features of Treacher Collins syndrome. *Ultrasound Obstet Gynecol* 19:414–415.

Tegnander E, Williams W, Johansen OJ, Blaas HG, Eik-Nes SH. 2006. Prenatal detection of heart defects in a non-selected population of 30,149 fetuses—detection rates and outcome. *Ultrasound Obstet Gynecol* 27:252–265.

Timor-Tritsch IE, Monteagudo A, Mayberry P. 2000. Three-dimensional ultrasound evaluation of the fetal brain: the three horn view. *Ultrasound Obstet Gynecol* 16:302–306.

Tonni G, Lituania M. OmniView algorithm. 2012. A novel 3-dimensional sonographic technique in the study of the fetal hard and soft palates. *J Ultrasound Med* 31:313–318.

Turan S, Turan OM, Ty-Torredes K, Harman CR, Baschat AA. 2009. Standardization of the first-trimester fetal cardiac examination using spatiotemporal image correlation with tomographic ultrasound and color Doppler imaging. *Ultrasound Obstet Gynecol* 33:652–656.

Turan S, Turan OM, Desai A, Harman CR, Baschat AA. 2014. A prospective study of first trimester fetal cardiac examination using spatiotemporal image correlation, tomographic ultrasound and color Doppler imaging for the diagnosis of complex congenital heart disease in high-risk patients. *Ultrasound Obstet Gynecol* ePub Mar 1.

Uittenbogaard LB, Haak MC, Spreeuwenberg MD, van Vugt JM. 2009. Fetal cardiac function assessed with four-dimensional ultrasound imaging using spatiotemporal image correlation. *Ultrasound Obstet Gynecol* 33:272–281.

United Healthcare. 2013. Clinical Policy. Obstetrical Sonography. https://www.oxhp.com/secure/policy/obstetrical_ultrasonography.pdf.

Varvarigos E, Iaccarino M, Iaccarino S, Mucerino J. 2002. Transabdominal multiplanar scan vs. B-mode in examination of fetal physiologic brain sagittal scan. *Ultrasound Obstet Gynecol* 20:84.

Verwoerd-Dikkeboom CM, Koning AHJ, Groenenberg IAL, Smit BJ, Brezinka C, Van Der Spek PJ, Steegers EAP. 2008. Using virtual reality for evaluation of fetal ambiguous genitalia. *Ultrasound Obstet Gynecol* 32:510–514.

Viñals F, Poblete P, Giuliano A. 2003. Spatio-temporal image correlation (STIC): a new tool for the prenatal screening of congenital heart defects. *Ultrasound Obstet Gynecol* 22:388–394.

Viñals F, Muñoz M, Naveas R, Shalper J, Giuliano A. 2005. The fetal cerebellar vermis: anatomy and biometric assessment using volume contrast imaging in the C-plane (VCI-C). *Ultrasound Obstet Gynecol* 26:622–627.

Viñals F, Ascenzo R, Poblete P, Comas C, Vargas G, Giuliano A. 2006. Simple approach to prenatal diagnosis of transposition of the great arteries. *Ultrasound Obstet Gynecol* 28:22–25.

Viñals F, Muñoz M, Naveas R, Giuliano A. 2007. Transfrontal three-dimensional visualization of midline cerebral structures. *Ultrasound Obstet Gynecol* 30:162–168.

Viora E, Sciarrone A, Bastonero S, Errante G, Botta G, Campogrande M. 2002. Three-dimensional ultrasound evaluation of short-rib polydactyly syndrome type II in the second trimester: a case report. *Ultrasound Obstet Gynecol* 19:88–91.

Vohra N, Rochelson B, Smith-Levitin M. 2003. Three-dimensional sonographic findings in congenital (Harlequin) ichthyosis. *J Ultrasound Med* 22:737–739.

Volpe P, Buonadonna AL, Campobasso G, Di Carlo A, Stanziano A, Gentile M. 2004. Cat-eye syndrome in a fetus with increased nuchal translucency: three-dimensional ultrasound and echocardiographic evaluation of the fetal phenotype. *Ultrasound Obstet Gynecol* 24:485–487.

Volpe P, Contro E, DeMusso F, Ghi T, Farina A, Tempesta A, Volpe G, Rizzo N, Pilu G. 2012. Brainstem-vermis and brainstem-tentorium angles allow accurate categorization of fetal upward rotation of cerebellar vermis. *Ultrasound Obstet Gynecol* 39:632–635.

Votino C, Cos T, Abu-Rustum R, Dahman Sidi S, Gallo V, Dobrescu O, Dessy H, Jani J. 2013. Spatio-temporal image correlation (STIC) modality at 11–14 weeks' gestation. *Ultrasound Obstet Gynecol* 42:669–678.

Wong HS, Parker S, Tait J, Pringle KC. 2008. Antenatal diagnosis of anophthalmia by three-dimensional ultrasound: a novel application of the reverse face view. *Ultrasound Obstet Gynecol* 32:103–105.

Wong HS, Tait J, Pringle KC. 2009. Examination of the secondary palate on stored 3D ultrasound volumes of the fetal face. *Ultrasound Obstet Gynecol* 33:407–411.

Yamamoto M, Essaoui M, Nasr B, Malek N, Takahashi Y, Moreira de Sa R, Ville Y. 2007. Three-dimensional sonographic assessment of fetal urine production before and after laser surgery in twin-to-twin transfusion syndrome. *Ultrasound Obstet Gynecol* 30:972–976.

Yeo L, Romero R. 2013. Fetal intelligent navigation echocardiography (FINE): a novel method for rapid, simple, and automatic examination of the fetal heart. *Ultrasound Obstet Gynecol* 42:268–284.

Youssef A, Bellussi F, Montaguti E, Maroni E, Salsi G, Maria Morselli-Labate A, Paccapelo A, Rizzo N, Pilu G, Ghi T. 2013. Agreement between two and three-dimensional methods for the assessment of the fetal head-symphysis distance in active labor. *Ultrasound Obstet Gynecol* 43:183–188.

Zalel Y, Yagel S, Achiron R, Kivilevich Z, Gindes L. 2009. Three-dimensional ultrasonography of the fetal vermis at 18 to 26 weeks' gestation time of appearance of the primary fissure. *J Ultrasound Med* 28:1–8.

Zheng Y, Zhou XD, Zhu YL, Wang XL, Qian YQ, Lei XY, Chen BL, Yu M, Xin XY. 2008. Three- and 4-dimensional ultrasonography in the prenatal evaluation of fetal anomalies associated with trisomy 18. *J Ultrasound Med* 27:1041–1051.

Zoppi MA, Ibba RM, Axiana C, Monni G. 2008. Prenatal sonographic features of isolated cleft soft palate with anterior axial three-dimensional view reconstruction. *Ultrasound Obstet Gynecol* 31:476–477.

INDEX

Note: Page references in **bold** refer to the Tables